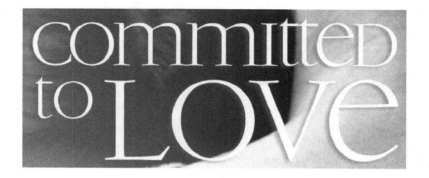

Committed to Love

By

Susan Lee Mintz

In the memory of Dr. Jeffrey A. Mintz.

30% of the proceeds will go directly to pay for
HIV/AIDS medications for persons not able to afford them.

Purpose Publishing
1503 Main Street #168 ♃ Grandview, Missouri
www.purposepublishing.com

Editing by Felicia Murrell
Book Cover Design by Lapridos Mairito

Preface

My book entitled *Committed to Love* is a deeply personal one. It explores the details of many issues and experiences I had to face in my marriage to a bisexual man who died of AIDS. It contains twenty-four chapters with personal stories and issues ranging from his diagnosis on June 19, 1992, with pneumonia and full blown AIDS to his death on August 17, 1994. I've spoken extensively in South Florida on living and coping with AIDS and other terminal or life threatening illnesses. In this particular area, I feel I make the most powerful impact. I am well acquainted with the devastation of AIDS, having lost my beloved husband of twenty-five years to this horrific disease. My marriage was unconventional and it was difficult. But, I would do it all over again because my journey with Jeff provided me the opportunity to discover my own true definition of love.

For many of us, thoughts of love evoke images of champagne, roses, and chocolates. For me, however, love has always meant commitment, unconditional acceptance and action. As an active resident of Boca Raton, Florida, I abide by my philosophy. I've done extensive charity and volunteer work with Hospice and the Comprehensive AIDS Program (CAP) of Palm Beach County. I've been a gourmet cook and author of a widely acclaimed cookbook. I've donated a large percentage of the sales from my book to both organizations. And I take great pride in the fact that I was an eleventh hour volunteer for Hospice and was called in to be with a family when a loved one's death was imminent.

Troy, New York –
The Journey Begins 1957

I met Jeffrey A. Mintz in the fifth grade in Troy, New York. I remember he looked at me and said, "I like your bobby socks." I was only eleven years old, a stranger in a new school. He made me feel accepted. I knew then there was a connection. At that very moment, I knew there was something special about him. We began an incredible friendship that endured throughout grammar school, high school and college. I was, however, not prepared for the events that followed.

I was a dental hygienist living in Boston and had come back home to Troy to marry someone else. Jeff had come back home from Springfield, Massachusetts to complete his Master's Degree at Albany State in Educational Psychology. One passionate encounter on a very special evening led to an unexpected pregnancy. It was 1968. Abortion was not legal. It was a small town. Jeff did what was right and expected. We told our parents and a subsequent marriage ensued. A week later while at work at the VA Hospital in Albany, I started to abort. I was taken to the doctor and later that evening on Jeff's 22nd birthday, I miscarried. No one ever knew I was pregnant except our family. I know now that it was our strong bond of friendship and caring that got me through this difficult time.

With the initial cause of marriage no longer an issue, we were at a crossroads. As I remember, we looked at each other and said, "Well, let's see what we can do." We tried because we cared. We always had a passion for each other and there was chemistry. He was my best friend. I loved and adored him. Four months later, my devotion was put to another test. On our honeymoon in Spain, Jeff confessed to me that he thought he was bisexual. He had a desire for men in his life. I remember thinking, *I am twenty-two years old. I've been married four months, and my husband thinks he is gay.* I was in a living nightmare. Still commitment prevailed and we managed to find a way to make our marriage and friendship work.

As careers dictated, in 1971 we moved to Gainesville, Florida where Jeff received his Doctorate Degree in Special Education. Then, in 1974, we moved to Houston. He then set up a private practice and his own management consulting company. Our final move was to Boca Raton in 1985. Through the years, our unique relationship endured its share of hardships, as well as great times. So many times, I screamed out loud, "As a marriage, it was difficult. As a friendship, it was perfect." Common goals, shared values, and a sense of fun and adventure held us together during the most trying periods of our life.

However, it was the next incident that would consequently alter the course of my entire life. In 1981, while watching a news program, the topic of AIDS was discussed. I was frozen in my body. The so-called "Gay Men's Disease" was taking young men's lives in San Francisco. I knew at that very moment, I had the reason why I was to stay with my husband and love him. I fought so hard not to think that this disease could happen to my Jeff, but I knew in my heart of hearts, that one day it would. He had been so promiscuous with so many lovers.

My only choice to protect myself was celibacy. Instead of wallowing in self-pity about my circumstances, I channeled my energies into piano playing, bodybuilding, and writing my cookbook. In keeping with my commitment to Jeff and our marriage, we remained intimate at all other levels and managed to stay together.

The years went by. We had our friendship, our security, and our denial that we had such issues and problems. Anything and everything can be put into a compartment that fits. We had our secrets well hidden from the public. On June 19, 1992, Jeffrey was diagnosed with Pneumocystis Carinii Pneumonia, PCP or full-blown AIDS. While at his bedside for two weeks, I could only watch him fight for life. He lay so gravely ill. I started to document his ordeal and never stopped writing during this insanity. My writing saved me. I have recorded every detail of this period of time in fifteen journals. My emotions were rampant. Rage, denial, hate, resentment, love, sadness, chaos. My toughest job was to have to tell his parents, our families, and our friends that Jeff had AIDS and how he acquired it. I could lie no more. The truth was all we had left.

I wrote in my journal, "My husband is a perfectionist. He has kept his private life private...We keep secrets everyday and our secrets will destroy us." Family and friends continued to support us. We felt love, compassion, and loyalty. After two weeks in the hospital, Jeffrey returned home. We danced under a full moon on July 4, 1992. We held each other under the stars on our balcony. He was so weak, so fragile. But, he was home. His pneumonia was gone. For the next six to eight months he rallied, though he never again would be one hundred percent. As the disease ran its course, it took its toll on both of us. Every aspect of our lives changed. We made plans. We tried to keep things as normal as possible. However, nothing was normal. Our entire life revolved around medications, doctor's appointments, lab work, x-rays, and so on and so on. One minute we had theater tickets and five minutes later he was so violently ill, he had to be carried to the bathroom.

I left no stone unturned, trying anything to restore my husband's health. We went from conventional to unconventional. We had the resources to get the best. The finest doctors, the newest drugs, vitamins, juicing, acupuncture, homeopathy, and any other thing we could find to keep Jeff alive. I went with him to every x-ray, every lab test, and every doctor's appointment. We were together constantly. His illness was my life. My world was crumbling slowly before my eyes. I wanted to die with him, but I couldn't. I had to live and stay strong and healthy because I was his support. Life support to his eventual death. As I held him in my arms so many times night after night, he would convulse from the spiked 105-degree temperatures that accompanied the illnesses associated with AIDS. I changed the sheets at 3:00 AM because his night sweats left him in a pool of water and drenched clothing. It was a movie. The movie was from hell.

Lovingly and unconditionally, I honored the vows I'd made at the age of twenty-two. My husband died on August 17, 1994, as he lived, with pride, with love, with dignity and with his best friend and family at his side. He died at home, surrounded by the artwork, the music, and the treasures he collected having extensively traveled around the world. I was at his side holding his hand and loving him when he took his last breath. Hospice was with me to give support when I lost my love.

I am very philosophical when I reflect back on this experience. I made a commitment to Jeffrey. That's the most important part of the whole thing. I just wish I could let people know how fulfilling it is to believe in something. You can live with adversity and not become vengeful. He and I had something that was worth fighting for, loving for, and dying for. I have no regrets. I take pride that I completed this mission. I made a 360-degree completion in my life. I tied up my twenty-five-year marriage into a neat package. I can live and go on with that. My husband never knew a day when he wasn't loved. I only offer this small bit of advice. If you make a commitment to love, LOVE. I hope that I will continue to live as I have believed.

Susan Lee Mintz

Table of Contents

"August 17, 1994
I Said Goodbye with the Words but
Not with My Heart"

1 Honeymoon in Spain

May 1999

Dear Jeff,

Another warm spring evening is drawing to a close. The sun is setting and a blazing crimson sky is appearing before my eyes. How many times have I watched this magnificent spectacle from our balcony? You always commented that sundown was my favorite part of the day. I remember you laughing as I told you how every sunset was the most beautiful one of all. You'd say, "Bee, I think this is the only time you're at peace with yourself." Jeff, where did the past five years go? I can still see your body being taken from our home on August 17th, 1994. I remember how you suffered during those two horrible years. It took me a long time to come to terms with your death, but I think you'd be proud of me. My broken heart has finally mended and though my new life still feels strange and awkward at times, I've moved on. Now, I only see your beautiful face and hear your soft sweet voice echoing in my ears. I said "goodbye, my love" on that day with the words on my lips, but not with my heart. I'll always cherish the memories of our twenty-five years together.

Jeff, tonight's sunset has me agitated and restless. I feel like electricity is surging through my body. My heart is racing and my hands are tingling. The sky looks like it's painted with blood. What's happening to me? Why am I so afraid? I closed my eyes to shut out the sky, but I continued to see the blood. It was slowly oozing down the mortally wounded animal's side. He was dying in front of me. I opened my eyes and I was in Malaga, Spain at a bullfight. It was April 1969. We were sitting in a stadium with a frenzied crowd cheering around us expressing their delight in the matador's victory. The brilliantly costumed bullfighter had challenged the beast and won. We stared amazed and overwhelmed at the performance we had just witnessed. Only the fans knew what would happen next.

I heard you laugh but was oblivious to my fate. You were laughing because you saw the matador look our way. You shrieked, "Bee, watch out!" You always called me Bee when you wanted to get my attention. Suddenly, I felt something warm and wet graze the left side of my face. It was rough and scratchy as it brushed against my cheek. The matador had cut the dead bull's ear off and thrown it into the crowd. I told you that day I wanted a souvenir, but a bloody hairy bull's ear was not what I had expected. That was just the beginning of my many unexpected surprises wasn't it, Jeff? Twenty-four hours earlier from our hotel balcony in Malaga, you confessed to your bride of four months your darkest secret. Nothing could've prepared me for what you told me that day. During one terrible argument, you'd put our already shaky marriage on the line and changed the next twenty-five years of our life.

I called you "Christopher Columbus" because you loved to travel. In high school, you'd go to Florida for Christmas vacation or spring break. In college, you'd go skiing in Colorado or sunning in Puerto Rico. When you'd tell me of your adventurous plans, your enthusiasm made me want to run away with you. After we got married, you wanted to take me somewhere exotic for our honeymoon. Between your teaching position in Albany and my job as a dental hygienist at the Veterans Administration Hospital, we were doing well for a couple of young kids. You joined the Jewish Teacher's Association of America because you wanted to travel. Every city in the world appealed to you and we could afford to go anywhere. Their prices were so inexpensive. After six weeks of intense deliberation, you finally chose the Costa del Sol of Spain. Our two weeks cost us $198.00. Remember the night your parents told us that their friends, including your godparents, were taking the same trip? Oh how we laughed every time we thought about four other couples "chaperoning" us around Spain. They didn't know the circumstances concerning our "quickie" marriage. How did we keep the pregnancy and my miscarriage a secret? To them, we were newlyweds going on our dream honeymoon to the Mediterranean.

We flew from New York to Madrid. I remember the ride to our hotel in Torremolinos was spectacular. Our room overlooked the turquoise and blue Mediterranean water and the hotel grounds were picturesque. It was the most beautiful place I'd ever seen. We spent the first few days enjoying deliciously unfamiliar foods in fascinating local restaurants. We made love everywhere. I was sexually attracted to you from the moment we met. I loved kissing and holding you. Running my fingers through your thick, dark, hair excited me. I told everyone I was in love with the fifth Beetle. Your white sparkling teeth and beautiful smile captured my heart. Your body was naturally muscular and perfectly proportioned. You had the gracefulness of a dancer and the handsome good looks of a movie star. To me, you were the most exciting man in the world.

We went shopping for days. You wanted to buy paintings, while I purchased a dozen pair of shoes. We weren't sure how much "stuff" we could take back to Albany and cram into a studio apartment. And "the troops" were constantly with us. They kept a safe distance and gave us our space, but we ate dinner, attended the shows, and took the tours together. We were two kids running wild in a foreign country and it was absolutely wonderful. We were beginning to think that our "rocky start" was finally over.

We spent the second week in Malaga. Our new hotel room was more beautiful than the one before. But, you'd changed during the trip. You became distant and I was uncomfortable around you. There was an underlying current that something wasn't right between us. From the beginning of our marriage, this feeling went beyond our hasty wedding, my pregnancy, and the miscarriage. We were lying together in a hammock on the balcony watching the sunset. Only inches apart from one another, yet I felt alone and uneasy. I can't remember how the quarrel started, but things quickly got out of hand. You hated to argue. You were soft-spoken, even-tempered, and sensitive. When you did yell, I'd laugh because you'd start to cough and your throat would get sore. I was the fighter, easily frustrated, violently angry, and viciously cruel. I lashed out at you shouting, "I know you only married me because I was pregnant." You screamed back, "I don't think I can really love anyone." I said, "Jeff, why are you so guarded, spoiled, and selfish? One minute you tell me you love me and want our marriage to work and then you say you don't. What keeps you so far away from me? Who are you, Jeff?"

I was relentless, pushing you for more and more. Finally, you said, "I think I'm gay. I've had men in my life sexually. I don't know what I am!" I froze. My tears turned to ice. What had I heard? "What do you mean you think your gay? You're so handsome, so perfect, and you've always dated beautiful girls in high school and college. I've never seen you without a girlfriend. I'd get jealous when I saw you with someone else. What do you mean?" You couldn't control your tears. You cried. Oh! How hard you cried. My heart was in my throat. I ran to the bathroom and threw up. This nightmare couldn't be happening. We stared at each other like two total strangers in disbelief.

I finally said, "First, I get pregnant. Then, we get married. I lose our baby on your birthday, and just when I think we might make this marriage work, you tell me you think you're gay." You said, "I've had two encounters with young men and I don't know what I am! I always dated and had sex with girls, but I've also had men." I asked you the same questions over and over again, "Are you bisexual? Are you homosexual? Do you want a divorce? What do we tell our parents? Is it because you were adopted? Is it because you think you weren't loved at birth by your biological parents?" I continued to ask you questions you didn't have any answers for.

We went through hours of hell, until we reached the point of exhaustion. The last thing I remember was falling asleep in your arms. As the sun came up in this storybook setting, a new day was before us. We woke up drained from the previous night's events. My eyes were swollen and half-closed, but as I looked over at you, I loved you. I wanted everything to go away. This was a bad dream. I wanted to believe last night didn't happen. You were my perfect man lying

SUSAN MINTZ | 22

next to me. I couldn't have this in my life. I wouldn't accept it. I convinced myself I could make you happy. Love conquers all. You thought you could change and maybe you really weren't gay. We were so naïve, but perhaps our inexperience and youth worked to our advantage. We were more afraid to be without each other than to stay together. Were the things we had in common enough to give this marriage and our friendship another try?

By 11:00 A.M., we had pulled ourselves together and met up with the group. By 1:00 P.M., we were enjoying the bullfight and had put the horror of the past night behind us. No one ever suspected a thing. We wanted to make it work. We always tried to give our marriage another chance. We cared about each other. That was the foundation for our entire relationship. You didn't change and my love didn't conquer all. But, you loved me in your own special way.

Though the evening air is warm, I'm so cold. The blood red sky has disappeared and the darkness surrounds me. It's been a long time since I've thought about Spain. Now, I want to take my memories and hide from them. I need to get away from the emptiness I feel. I'll crawl into bed and pull the covers tightly around my body. The last thing I remember seeing before I drifted off to sleep was the matador and the bull. The skilled matador had won his battle this time. My darling Jeff, the beast you fought was AIDS and you didn't win your fight. Good Night, My Darling.

2 The Fear Factor

1971-1981

Dear Jeff,

What a beautiful day June 19th, 1971, was. You completed your Master's Degree in Educational Psychology from Albany State University on schedule. Those two years weren't easy, were they? You didn't like studying and I hated my dental hygiene job at the Veterans Administration Hospital. Our proud parents beamed as you walked down the aisle to receive your diploma. Now we had to decide where to go for your doctorate degree. Remember our trip around the country to check out the universities? You finally decided on the University of Florida in Gainesville. You wanted to get your Doctorate in Special Education with emotionally disturbed children and I'd get licensed as a dental hygienist. It was August 1st, 1971. We packed up our belongings, said good-bye to our parents, and together we followed our dream. You wanted to become Dr. Jeffrey A. Mintz.

Jeff, you tried to convince yourself you weren't gay. I know you were faithful to me during our two years in Albany. When you said you wanted our marriage to work and you were straight, I believed you. Why shouldn't I? You were young and questioned your sexuality just as I did. I was angry and frustrated. I initiated most of our arguments. They weren't about adjusting to newly married life. My problems were more complicated and I didn't want to face them.

Why was I so susceptible to urinary tract and vaginal yeast infections? I couldn't continue to blame the miscarriage for everything. You knew how much I hated going to the doctor's office, getting examined, and taking medications for weeks at a time. I was miserable, uncomfortable, and I resented you for causing my distress. I began to think that sexual intercourse was more of a detriment than a pleasure. But, these infections were just the beginning of my sexual problems with you. Later on, several other diseases came along affecting our sexual relationship. The choices I made to safeguard my health ultimately saved my life.

We weren't prepared for the difficulties and problems we'd encounter during the next three years. Gainesville wasn't the cosmopolitan dynamic city we'd anticipated. We loved the warm tropical climate of Florida, but it wasn't the city of our dreams. Remember that Monday morning when I answered the phone and was told the dentist I worked for had been burned in a fire? Now I was unemployed and we were living on your fellowship. It wasn't easy scaling back on an already limited budget. Eventually, I found work at the university answering the phone for the maintenance department. What a fulfilling career that was for a future doctor's wife. During our first year in Florida, you tried to be "straight", but it was hard. There was an active gay community in Gainesville and you wanted "your other life." You told me you were studying late, but I knew about the man you were meeting in the library. How many lovers did you have during the next two years? What did it matter? I didn't trust you any longer and I resented your lies and infidelity. But, I couldn't leave you. I focused on that degree and did whatever it took to help you achieve it. We also couldn't give up on each other.

Even with all our problems, baby, we had fun. How many times did we anxiously await our parents' visits? We'd laugh because they were always a bit shaky after their shuttle flight from Jacksonville to Gainesville. In between our quarterly semester breaks, we'd drive to Atlanta, Orlando, Savannah, or New Orleans. You planned the most wonderful adventures to new and exciting cities. And we loved the warm wonderful weather compared to Albany. We'd go to the beach every weekend. We rode our bikes to the *Gator* football games and ate lots of pizza. We faced financial problems, fought continuously about your *late nights out,* and dealt with many stressful situations. But, on June 15th, 1974, you became Dr. Jeffrey A. Mintz, Ed.D. It was the most exciting summer of my life and all our dreams had come true. I was married to the handsomest, most successful man in the world. Everything was going to turn out all right after all. Wasn't it, Jeff?

We left Gainesville on August 15th, 1974, ready to start a new life in Houston, Texas, the sixth largest city in the country. We were impressed with its wealth, flamboyance, and Tex-Mex culture. Your job as director of a well-known youth treatment and residential facility for emotionally disturbed children was an incredible opportunity. Do you remember how hard I tried to find a patient for the clinical part of my Texas dental hygiene boards? I combed the streets for two days looking for someone who desperately needed their teeth cleaned. I worked part-time because we wanted to buy our first home. I called you my "princess" because you enjoyed every comfort known to man. The word "Queen" was never an appropriate one for you. You loved great food, fine dining, exciting vacations, beautiful clothes, and *shopping*. I was the frugal and thrifty one. You wanted to spend money. I wanted to save it. But, when it came to our family and friends, we never thought twice. We had our priorities straight and lacked for nothing. We started traveling and collecting art and paintings from our numerous trips. We enjoyed our good fortune. But, we couldn't escape our problems. In fact, our problems were just beginning.

In 1975, we built our first home in a suburban Houston community. We decided we weren't going to have children and adopted a six-week old Schnauzer instead. We laughed for days trying to decide on a name that went with Mintz. Finally, we chose *Spear*. He was our baby for fourteen years. Jeff, isn't it ironic how I'd slept with dozens of men before

SUSAN MINTZ | 30

you and didn't get pregnant? We had sex once and I conceived. I lost the baby six weeks later and never got pregnant again. Why do you think I got pregnant, Jeff? Was it fate or destiny, my love? Do you think it was just supposed to happen?

The two and a half years we lived in our home, I was happier than I'd ever been. But, you didn't feel the same way. You hated the traffic commuting into downtown Houston. You thought living in suburbia was boring and yard work wasn't your form of leisure time activity. But the real reason you hated living outside the city was because your other *life* was in town, not in the suburbs. It was difficult for you to be with your male lovers, to go to the bars, and the bathhouses. So, in 1978, you found us a beautiful old townhouse in the *artsy* Montrose area of Houston. With its different ethnic cultures, shops, and restaurants, you loved feeling like you were in the middle of everything. I hated the house, the area, and the *gay element* around us. Did you know I was never jealous of your lovers? They never posed any threat to me. And I never worried about other women. What I hated was my weakness and inability to leave you and the co-dependent relationship we'd established. Why weren't we strong enough to get out of this marriage? You're the one who wanted the men in your life. I could've accepted the friendship and the security you were providing me. What were we so afraid of?

I remember when I made my decision to stay married to you. It was in 1981, while listening to the evening news. I'd taken Spear for a walk and was making dinner. It was 6:30 PM and Peter Jennings began his commentary about "The Gay Men's Disease" that was surfacing in San Francisco. He said, "Health agencies in San Francisco and Atlanta were becoming increasingly aware that gay men were getting seriously ill with an immune deficiency disorder called AIDS. It was deadly and there was no cure. Men in a high-risk category included homosexuals, intravenous drug users sharing needles, and blood contact with someone already infected with HIV." HIV was the name given to the virus responsible for the disease they were calling AIDS.

The report wasn't extensive since little information was known. This *plague* had the potential to spread and kill thousands or millions of people. One theory stated it originated in Africa. Did humans, animals, or a mosquito transmit it? Did this deadly virus come from a government lab? Were we the unsuspecting victims of a cover-up? Or could it be blamed on the gay community, the prostitutes, and the drug users? No one knew very much about this "killer virus." But I didn't need facts and figures. At that moment, I knew all I needed to know about AIDS. You were in the high-risk category. You were a homosexual practicing unsafe sex with numerous partners for many years.

I was terrified and wanted to faint. Gripped in terror, I was perspiring and frozen at the same time. How could I compose myself and tell you about this? Did you already know about this deadly disease? Several of my dental patients had been taken to the hospital recently and passed away. I was told one died from cancer and another from pneumonia. A few men at my hair salon had also taken ill and died. It happened to several men in our neighborhood too. Was the report correct? Oh, Jeffrey! This couldn't happen to you. You didn't fit the profile of a gay man who could die from this rare and unknown disease. You were married, healthy, and exercised. I was an incredible cook and took great care of you. I tried to rationalize everything. But in my heart of hearts, I knew why it would be "till death do us part", my darling.

You came home around 8:00 PM. I knew something was terribly wrong. I didn't say anything as I wrapped my arms tightly around you. Spear was jumping up and down barking excitedly because *Daddy* was home. The three of us were standing at the door, wrapped up in each other's arms. We were a family who shared a special life. My world, my future, and everything I loved were all together in a small 360-degree circle. I took your hand and said "Jeff, I need to talk to you. I'm scared and don't know what to do." You put your briefcase down and walked to the couch. How I loved your sweet and gentle nature. You looked straight into my eyes and said, "Susan, are you sick?" I wanted to laugh at the irony. I was going to ask you about a deadly virus and you thought I was the one who was ill.

I started to shake. You took my hands and said, "Susan, please tell me what's wrong. What's going on? You're scaring me." I said, "Jeff, have you heard of AIDS? Have you heard of a disease that's killing gay men? Have you known anyone that's died from it? Have you been sexually active with any man who's been ill? Jeff, how do you feel?" I asked you a dozen questions, one after another. I wanted to purge my body of these thoughts. You looked at me with those beautiful brown eyes and said quietly, "Yes, I've heard of HIV and AIDS. I've recently known several men who have taken ill with pneumonia and have died. Yes, Susan, I know of AIDS." I said, "Jeff, what are we going to do? You're bisexual. You've had sex with many men. You could become ill and die. You must get tested. You can't wait."

You never got emotional or upset. You hugged me for a long time and finally said something I'll never forget as long as I live. You said, "Susan, this will never happen to me. When I have intercourse, no man ejaculates in me. I'm not the one who gets penetrated. I have mostly oral sex and masturbation. Besides, you're my protector. As long as I have you, nothing will go wrong. I'm not going to get ill and we'll grow old together." Jeff, you always believed I could work miracles and your trust in me was frightening. But, I think you went into denial and the only way you could handle this issue was to place the emphasis on me. I knew in 1981, that I'd bury you, my true love and soul mate from this horrible disease. Another thirteen years passed before my premonition came true.

3 Chosing Celibacy to Protect Myself

1974-1985

Dear Jeff,

Do you know how many times I questioned my sanity? I had to be crazy to be living like this. I thought I must have done something terrible as a child and this was the way I punished myself. Did you know for years I thought that I was the only woman in the world who was married to a bisexual? I didn't know there were millions of couples living lifestyles similar to ours. Why did I choose to live a life that presented so many obstacles? My darling, I wish the answer wasn't so simple. Why? Because I thrived on it. My life with you was energy and passion. My life with you was life. I was a hurricane that gained strength over the warm waters our relationship provided. My life was a roller coaster ride but I didn't want to get off. When I was up, I was in heaven. And when I was down, I was in hell. The ride made vicious sharp turns and threw my body from side to side. I'd squeal with joy one minute and be brought to tears the next. Our marriage challenged me as I was presented with decisions most people might never have to make. Maybe my life was totally out of control but, it was my life. Maybe I was strong, crazy or a little of both.

We knew after I lost the baby that we weren't going to have any children. Getting pregnant was the catalyst that brought us together, but we weren't supposed to be parents. It wasn't because we were selfish. We just didn't want to admit that we couldn't have made the sacrifices involved with raising kids. Having children wasn't going to fit into our lifestyle. How could we bring a child into our unstable environment? I'd been taking birth control pills since the miscarriage and began to experience some side effects from their long-term use. After seven years of marriage, we'd stopped having sex as frequently as we had before. The spontaneity and passion had dwindled over the years and we weren't doing anything to rekindle those dying embers. We knew that Houston was going to be our home for a long time. We'd built our house, you had a wonderful job you enjoyed, and I had time to do the things I'd always wanted to do. On May 4th, 1976, my thirtieth birthday, you came home from work with flowers, cards, and my favorite perfume. Then you said to me, "Susan, this is a special birthday. We'll do anything you want to do." I said, "Jeff, I'd like to get my tubes tied. I want to check into the hospital, buy a sexy nightgown, and get fixed."

You didn't expect that, did you? It was a difficult decision for us to make, but it was the right one. My doctor said the insurance company wouldn't pay for the procedure. I was thirty years old, didn't have any medical reason for the surgery, and I might change my mind and want children later on. On a personal level, my doctor didn't have any problems performing the operation. She believed it was my right to decide what was best for me. She told us that if I had a psychological reason for the surgery, they would approve it. I told her you were bisexual and we chose to stay married. Children wouldn't fit into our family picture. I think it was the quickest letter ever drafted to an insurance company. The ink was still wet when she mailed it to them. I was scheduled two weeks later for my tubal ligation. After the operation, I remember coming out of the anesthesia and telling her I thought the psychological factor made the whole thing even more dramatic and exciting. You said to her, "Susan never has a problem with the difficult decisions. It is always the little ones that throw her."

When we were first married, I blamed you for my frequent vaginal infections. I knew they weren't your fault, but I was miserable. I didn't enjoy having sex because I was afraid of getting another yeast infection. Eventually, I accepted the fact that I was prone to getting them whether we had sex or not. In 1978, two years after I'd had my tubes tied, you gave me the first sexually transmitted disease. It was syphilis. I had a sore around my genital area that wouldn't go away. After two weeks, I went to my gynecologist. She said I had syphilis. I didn't know how to react. I said, "Syphilis! How could that be? Only dirty people get syphilis. No, I can't have that." But, I did have syphilis and I got it from you. She gave me antibiotics, said the sore would go away, and that I would be fine. At that moment, hatred was the only feeling I had towards you. When you came home I said, "You gave this to me. How could you? You don't even know which one of your dirty partners gave you this disease. How could you be so careless with your body?" This was my wake-up call. It prepared me for other more terrifying diseases in the future.

A couple of years later, I'd experience the second sexually transmitted disease. This one was more serious and remained with me the rest of my life. It started with a burning and tingling in my vaginal area. Then, I experienced an increase in my vaginal secretions. I broke out with small blisters on my genitals. The next phase was a lesion that lasted seven to ten days. It was terribly painful. The outbreaks were several weeks apart but continuous. This went on for six months. I was afraid and didn't know what to do. When I mentioned this to you, you said you had the same thing once in a while. Other than my gynecologist, I didn't have anyone to talk to about these infections. I finally went to the doctor. She said it was genital herpes. I couldn't believe what I was hearing. She told me to take the anti-viral Zovirax regularly, watch my diet, and reduce the stress. How could I reduce the stress? I was stress. I hated you more and more. I confronted you screaming, "You bastard. You, filthy bastard. First, you gave me syphilis and now a virus I'll have for the rest of my life. How many more disgusting diseases are you going to give me?"

I referred to your partners as "The Generic Brand" because you met them in baths or bars. Many of them didn't even have a name. You had this amazing gift for using people, but you always made them feel good about it. I never wanted to know the details of your liaisons and desperately tried to erase your *nights out* from my thoughts. However, the diseases you gave me were from unprotected, unsafe sex with men you didn't know. You'd developed a sexual pattern of behavior with your lovers and the ensuing sexual relationships were based on one thing, these men satisfied your need to be with a man. No more, no less. It was lust and sex. It wasn't pretty. There weren't any commitments, and they never lasted. They were one night stands but I hated you for what you were doing to me. I was sick of being sick and tired of getting diseases from second hand partners. I was psychologically and physically scared to have sex because I didn't want to go through any more pain. I didn't care if you put a condom on. I didn't want you to touch me any longer. I was becoming frigid and the thought of sexual intercourse turned me off. I said to you, "If I want to get a disease, I'll get it first hand from my own partner, not yours." I knew I was going to have to take care of myself or I'd suffer more serious consequences.

In the early 80's with the AIDS epidemic increasing, so was the number of innocent lives lost to this deadly disease. When you told me you'd met someone *significant* I knew I had to make a life-altering decision. I couldn't allow myself to be put at risk any longer. I couldn't change you and I wouldn't leave you. Choosing celibacy was the only thing I could do to protect myself. I remember every detail when I told you my decision. We'd agreed that Tuesday and Thursday evenings would be your two nights out. Late one Friday evening, you called stating you wanted to see a *drag show* at a local gay bar. You said you wouldn't be home late. It was 4:00 AM when you finally came home. I was furious. How dare you use me and take advantage of our private time? When you got into bed, I turned on the light. You were surprised because you thought I was sleeping. I said, "Jeff, I'm only going to say this once. You are who you are and I'll try my best to accept that. I'll love you, live with you, and care for you. But, I won't die for you. I know you won't get an HIV test. Therefore, I won't have sexual intercourse with you any longer. Every time you have sex with a man, you're putting my life on the line, too. I have to take matters into my own hands. I've made this decision for my own protection." You were calm and understanding. You said, "I respect your decision and if that's your choice, I'll accept it." That was the end of our conversation. That decision saved my life.

I knew my commitment to love and stay with you was the right one. It was my choice and I've never regretted that decision. Looking back, why do you think I put myself through such mental and emotional abuse? I've asked myself that question a thousand times. The answer was always the same. I loved you, Jeff. I loved you because you were worth loving. There were times I didn't like you and sometimes I hated you. But, I never stopped loving you. I believed in us and I couldn't give up on you. You once told me, "Susan, you're the most stubborn, persistent, never give up, focused person I know. You're a true "Taurus the Bull." That was one of the greatest compliments you ever gave me. Do you remember your reward? I made you the best eggplant Parmesan you'd ever eaten. You may have wanted other men in bed, but I was the only one who could satisfy you in the kitchen.

June 19, 1992

Dear Jeff,

We were having dinner one evening and I said, "Jeff, you've never forgotten my birthday, our anniversary, or any other special occasion that gave us a reason to celebrate." You said, "Susan, certain dates become etched in your mind and you can't forget them no matter how hard you try." Over the years, we were very fortunate to have celebrated so many wonderful occasions with our family and friends. But, we knew a few tragic dates, didn't we? Dates that brought us great pain and sorrow. Yes, Jeff, there was one date I wish I could erase from my mind. It was a date so horrible and terrifying and it changed our life forever. On that date, I said good-bye to my life as I watched you fight desperately for yours. We were thrown upside down and everything we had become or ever wanted to be was over. We were living inside someone else's nightmare as we entered our own private hell. This frightening new life was ours. It was Friday, June 19th, 1992. I can still hear our doctor telling us you had Pneumocystis Carinii Pneumonia and AIDS. And now, my darling, five years after your death, I must tell you honestly how that terrible date in June changed the rest of my life. Your diagnosis opened the door to my future and in it, I would eventually find the peace and happiness I'd been searching for.

My poor Jeff, you hadn't been feeling well for so long. I was afraid because I knew what was happening. By now, it was the early 90's and the AIDS epidemic was ten years old. How many men had we known whose symptoms of HIV were similar to yours? Do you think I wanted to face the truth? Of course I didn't. And, I didn't have the courage to confront you about it. I wanted desperately to believe that my love for you was powerful enough to save you from this horrible fate. I tried to rationalize your symptoms, but every night for twelve months, I went to bed knowing that you were infected with this deadly virus. You denied their insidious and subtle warning signs. But, that was your nature. You never wanted to face yourself. You denied your homosexuality for years. You wouldn't go for an HIV test. And you couldn't tell your parents who loved you so much that you weren't the *perfect* son you wanted to be. You spent much of your life running from the truth about yourself. Now there was no place to run and nowhere to hide. Your past had finally caught up with you.

For twelve months, I watched your healthy magnificent body deteriorate. It started with your skin. Every aspect of it changed. You always had a dark glowing complexion that radiated vitality and good health. Your skin was dry and dull. In many lights, it looked yellow. For the first time in your life, you had dandruff. It was in your hair, around your eyebrows, the bridge of your nose and your mustache. You broke out with little pimples on your legs that itched constantly. You scratched them so intensely they bled. You tried every lotion and ointment, but nothing seemed to work. The next significant change came with your weight. I'd seen many people *waste away* from this disease, but now I saw it happening to you. From the beginning of our marriage, you weighed between 165-170 pounds. I envied your ability to eat anything you wanted and never gain a pound. Now, it continued to drop and your appetite diminished. You were chewing your food more slowly and taking deep breaths in order to finish a meal. However, my worst fears came at night. I couldn't sleep with you any longer. You were snoring. Your breathing was labored, and you were restless. You struggled for air, making sounds that frightened me. You weren't the man I'd known for twenty-three years. Everything about you was changing. If these changes were outwardly visible, what was happening inside your body?

In the beginning of June 1992, your fevers spiked to 103-104 degrees for several days. I had to change the sheets in the middle of the night because your *night sweats* drenched the bed. The chills accompanying the fevers were violent. You were having convulsions. Fearful that you would hurt yourself, I'd lie on top of you holding you down. You couldn't catch your breath and walking to the bathroom tired you out. And then there was that horrible cough. You suffered for weeks but blamed it on a sinus condition. Finally, we called our doctor. He said to come in immediately for a chest x-ray and blood work. When he saw you, he knew it was serious. The x-ray revealed pneumonia. He said that could be causing your symptoms because you could've had it for a while. He gave you an antibiotic and said he'd call us tomorrow with the lab reports. We were almost happy to hear it was only pneumonia. We waited anxiously for the results. You'd gotten worse overnight and couldn't breathe. At 5:00 PM on June 19th, 1992, the phone rang. Our doctor was downstairs. The look on his face said it all. I held your hand as he gave us the devastating news. Your AIDS test came back positive. He thought you had PCP pneumonia and full-blown AIDS. You'd be admitted into the hospital in the morning.

You were infected with a deadly virus that didn't have a cure. How could we handle the disease when we didn't know if we could cope with the diagnosis? What were our reactions that Friday in June? We felt shock, denial, disbelief, anger, fear, hate, relief, acceptance, and finally, hope. We went into shock and denied the words we'd just heard. We became angry because life was cruel and we wanted to blame others for our suffering. We questioned our doctor, the blood work, and the results. There must have been a mistake. We said he was wrong, that we would get a second opinion. But, there wasn't any mistake. After our doctor left, we collapsed in each other's arms. We held one another for hours, and cried ourselves to sleep. The next morning, we were going to fight the battle to save your life.

On Saturday, June 20th, 1992, you entered the hospital. You were so ill you didn't know what was happening. I was a zombie filling out forms I didn't read and signing documents I couldn't understand. You were immediately taken to isolation and ICU. I don't remember much else about that day. As your wife and best friend for twenty-three years, there was nothing I could do for you now. I stood by feeling helpless and hopeless as you fought for your life. And that, my love, was when I started to write in my journals. I took a piece of paper, a pen, and documented what I was seeing and feeling. I couldn't write fast enough. Tears streamed down my cheeks as I scribbled words I could barely read. I was numb. My nerves raw, my heart ached for you. I loved you more at that moment than ever. I had to capture my thoughts on paper or I'd go insane. I ran downstairs to the gift shop and bought a spiral bound notebook. It would be the first of fifteen journals I would write. My writing kept me focused, and became my chosen career after you died.

I wrote, "I questioned the doctors, the nurses, and the lab technicians. I doubted everything and didn't trust anyone. Who were all these strangers taking care of you? Why are they doing this to you? Everyone had something to do or some task to perform. Everyone but me. You were their patient, but I was your wife. I should be the one taking care of you. I'm the one who took charge of everything and stayed in control. I want to tell them to leave you alone because I won't allow you to die. My frustrations are overwhelming. I can't turn my mind off. I feel useless, like I'm on the outside looking in."

As I wrote down my thoughts those first few hours, I realized I'd never faced any medical emergency or crisis before. My parents didn't sit me down and say read this book. It will tell you everything you'll need to know about catastrophic illness. Where was the printed outline to follow that would guide me through my anguish? There wasn't anyone or anything that could've prepared me for the diagnosis of a life-threatening illness. And this disease had a stigma around it that other illnesses didn't have. People were afraid to come in contact with those infected with HIV. Even in 1992, little was known about this deadly virus and the mention of the word caused many to turn away. Therefore, how was I to feel? What was I to do? Who would be there for me? Where would I go for help? I knew I felt alone, isolated, and scared. The fear of the unknown consumed me. Though people were all around, there wasn't anyone who could hear my cries for help.

I wrote, "My worst fears have come true. I prayed you wouldn't become HIV positive and develop AIDS, but you did. Do you know how fearful I was every time you didn't feel well? Since 1981, I've lived in my own cocoon, a dark cloud hanging over my head. I faced my fears about your lifestyle and this dreaded disease alone. I rationalized every symptom. Who could I tell? I'd done everything in my power to protect myself and to keep you safe and well. As I write my feelings down, I'll call the next phase of my life, "My Fear Factor." Because it's the only thing I'm feeling now."

I watched and wrote for twenty-four hours as a constant stream of doctors, nurses, and clinicians went in and out of your room. All hours of the day and night, people were taking your vital signs, drawing blood, and hooking you up to monitors and machines. You were on oxygen, receiving fluids, and given several antibiotics to combat this deadly infection. Barely alive, you were unaware of the seriousness of your condition. If the doctors couldn't stabilize you, you would die. All you could do was fight to stay alive. Dazed and numb, I wanted to crawl up inside myself and hide. But, there was one more thing I had to do and it couldn't wait any longer. I had to tell your parents.

June 21, 1992

Dear Jeff,

I was standing outside your hospital room waiting for your parents to arrive. I was exhausted and thought I was going to faint. The wall was the only thing holding me up. One of your nurses came over and said, "You need a hug. Then you need to eat and get away from this room. You can't do anything for your husband now and he's going to need you later. You've got to take care of yourself. You've been carrying around a heavy burden for a long time. I'm terribly sorry about what you're going through, and I understand your pain. My brother died from AIDS two years ago. Everyone involved suffers with this disease." I started crying again. She brought over a box of tissues and shoved them under my arm. Her caring gesture made me smile. I said, "When I called Jeff's parents all I told them was that he had taken ill and was in the hospital. I asked them to please come immediately. We needed them. How could I tell them any more over the phone?" She said something to me I'll never forget. She said, "Susan, you might lose a husband, but they are going to lose a child." She understood how difficult this would be for everyone.

Jeff, did you know that our parents had been friends for forty years? When you were adopted, your parents sent mine the announcement. Troy was a small town and everyone in the Jewish community knew your parents wanted a child for a long time. One day your parents went to New York City and came back with a beautiful six-week old baby boy named Jeffrey Alan Mintz. You were the perfect child. I remember the first book we unpacked when we moved into our apartment. It was entitled "The Chosen Baby." Your rabbi gave it to your parents when they brought you home. I still have the book. You were the chosen baby who grew up to be a remarkable human being. The sun rose on your beautiful face and set on your gentle nature.

You were a wonderful son who adored your parents. You brought them such joy and pleasure. Your relationship with them was always special. I envied and admired it because I didn't have the communication and understanding with my parents growing up. You never argued, said anything unkind, or had any conflicts. After we got married, I knew I'd inherited two other parents. I respected the bond you had with them and never interfered or tried to compete. It would have been a futile battle. A parent's love is sacred and special. I knew as your wife what role I was to play and what part of you I could have. They loved me because I loved you, and they trusted me.

As ill as you were, you were able to tell me what you wanted. You asked me to call your parents and tell them what was happening and why. I dreaded making that call. But, if they wanted to see their son alive, I had to do it now. Jeff, as terrified as I was to tell your parents, another part of me was relieved. I'd wanted them to know for so long. But, why did they have to find out like this? If you had been honest with your parents, I'd have been able to share my feelings with the other woman who loved you as much as I did. Do you know how much I needed to talk to your mother about our life? I loved her, Jeff. She wasn't my mother-in-law. She was your mother. Therefore, she was mine. I hated you for deceiving them and I resented you for not allowing me to share my feelings with her. When I desperately needed a friend to talk to, she would've been there. When I questioned my marriage and my life with its complex and painful conditions, she would've listened.

You've given me some rough times and difficult challenges, but I don't know if I can do this? How are your parents going to be able to cope? How will I find the strength to tell them? Why did you wait until you were dying to give me this responsibility? Why did you need to be perfect? Why couldn't you have trusted your parent's love and have accepted yourself? I loved you no matter what you were. You had an unconditional love relationship with your parents. Nothing would've changed that. Had you been honest with yourself years ago, you could've spared everyone so much sorrow. Just last month we were all together having dinner. You looked wonderful and acted as if everything was perfect. They didn't know you hadn't been feeling well and they certainly never noticed any symptoms. Now, it's too late and you can't hide the truth from them. What do I say? "Mom and Dad, your son might die from a life-threatening illness that doesn't have a cure." When they ask me how you got AIDS, I can say, "Jeff is bisexual. He's had many affairs with men over the years and contracted this disease from having unsafe, unprotected sex." How do I tell your parent's this? It's Sunday, June 21st, 1992, Father's Day.

When I called, I chose my words carefully, giving them very little information over the phone. I could barely contain myself and didn't want to break down during our conversation. I told them you were ill and they should come immediately to the hospital. I gave them the directions and said I'd wait outside the room. As I watched your parents walk down the corridor, I fell apart. When they saw the terrible condition I was in, they knew something serious had happened. It was horrible, Jeff. Seeing them affected me more than I'd expected. I tried to keep myself together but couldn't. My heart ached for them. I couldn't look them in the eyes. My stomach was in my throat. I was shaking and crying hysterically, choking on my words. I wasn't making any sense. Finally, I reached out and took their hands. I held them so tightly. I put my arms around each of them hugging them as if they'd disappear within an instant. Through my tears and broken sounds I said, "Jeff has AIDS."

As they entered the room, you were delirious with a 104-degree fever. You were trying to rip the oxygen tube from your nose. A machine monitoring your vital signs was attached to your chest. Both arms had IV's coming out of them. One was a dextrose solution for dehydration and the other was an antibiotic for the pneumonia. There were gloves, masks, gowns, and supplies everywhere. You were in a private room, in isolation and your condition was guarded. There had been only one other AIDS patient on the floor during the past year. How this deadly virus was transmitted was of serious concern to everyone. People were being professional and performing their duties, but they were treating you like a leper. I understood their attitude but hated it. I'd lived with you for twenty-three years and I was healthy. Haven't you people heard? "You don't get AIDS from loving someone."

It was your parents' time to say I love you to their son. I was thankful we hadn't waited any longer. They'd arrived in time and you were alive. Though seeing you this way was difficult, it could've been worse. Oh, Jeff, if we were unprepared for this and in shock, how could they possibly comprehend the magnitude and gravity of this situation? What must your parents be thinking? Our marriage and life was centered around homosexuality. We were knowledgeable about AIDS and had known many that died. We knew you were at risk and might become HIV positive. However, until we heard the actual diagnosis, we were naïve to think we were prepared for this. We'd never be ready to hear those terrifying words. Only one thing was certain at this time. The four of us would face this crisis together and somehow manage to deal with it. We would support, comfort, and reassure each other.

All they wanted was to see their son. They wanted to touch you, to comfort you, to love you. Your mom spoke first. She said, "Jeff, your parents are here and we love you, honey." Dad said, "You're the best son in the world. You've done everything right. Just get better and live. Please, Jeff. You must fight to live." They wanted you to know you weren't alone. Your family was here. You had our love, respect, and acceptance. I was thankful they never asked me any questions. Why you were ill, how you got sick, or anything else that didn't matter now. On that Father's Day in June, all your parents wanted was to look at their son and be there for you.

It took several hours, but finally your fever came down. You looked at them and smiled. They desperately needed to see that beautiful smile reassuring them of their presence. I left the room because they needed their private time with you. I had other matters to attend to. Now, I had to tell my family and a few close friends. I didn't have the energy to call my parents. I'd ask my sister in Boston if she would handle it. When I called her, she broke down. Surprisingly enough, I was calm. She said she'd do anything she could and if I needed her, she would fly in. I told her, quite honestly, I didn't know who or what I needed. I decided to tell our friends that you were in the hospital with pneumonia. I said your condition was serious but you were stable. This information sufficed for now. After several calls, I felt relieved. A weight had finally been lifted from me. For the first time in twenty-three years, we would have to be honest about our marriage and our life. I felt so much support from our family and friends and was hopeful because I wouldn't have to be alone with my secrets any more.

Wednesday, June 24, 1992

Dear Jeff,

You've been in the hospital for five days. Your condition has stabilized and the doctor says you're doing well. For now, he thinks the crisis is over. It will take you a long time to regain your strength, but you're going to pull through. My writing has helped clear the cobwebs from my mind and it's given me something to focus on. Somebody once told me that writing was therapeutic, but I didn't understand how powerful that statement was until now. By being able to express my feelings on paper I've come to terms with a very difficult issue. It's one that has caused me years of pain and unhappiness. Through my writing, I've discovered something about myself that I'd never been willing to face before. I realized that I've spent much of my life being a *why me person*. I've allowed the *why me questions* and *why me person* to control me. For twenty-three years, three questions have frustrated and discouraged me. They've left me feeling helpless and hopeless. Why have they caused me such anguish? Because asking myself *why me questions* didn't have the answers to my problems. I had to change the way I looked at myself and *why* I was the way I was. That's when I became my own best friend and dealt with my life effectively. Once I understood that I was the problem, I was able to deal with it.

You better than anyone knew how much my life has always needed to make sense. Everything had to be in order, things had to fit properly, and nothing could ever be left to chance. What's happened because of my writing is I've discovered *my life needed to have a reason, but it didn't always have to make any sense*. Everything may not always be right and some questions will not have any answers. Sometimes things are just the way they are and that's the way it's supposed to be. For me to understand this was quite a revelation and recognizing it has brought me comfort and peace for the first time in my life. I couldn't do the *pity party* and *why me* any longer. If I didn't stop asking those unanswerable questions, I wouldn't be here with you now. On June 24th, 1992, "y" will be a letter in the alphabet not a word used in my life. From now on, I'll ask only *why not me* questions. They won't demand answers from me I cannot find nor cause the sadness I've brought on myself. As I sit here writing at your bedside, I'll share with you some of my *why me questions*. It's time to finally say good-bye to "The Why Me Factors" in my life.

The first *why me question*, I asked myself was *why did I get pregnant?* If this hadn't occurred, we wouldn't have gotten married. We weren't lovers in love. We were best friends who made love one night. During that brief encounter, our lives were changed forever. In 1969, we were two Jewish kids from a small conservative city, abortion wasn't legalized, and our families knew each other. Marriage was the only thing we could do. For the past twenty-three years, I've tried to understand the issue of *why did this happen to me?* But every time I asked myself *why me,* I became angry and resentful. I hated myself, but I hated you more. Most of my hostility towards you during those first few years was because I couldn't find any answers to the *why did I get pregnant* question. Now I say, *why not me* and I feel peaceful and calm. Why shouldn't this have happened? We knew it was a possibility. We had intercourse. I got pregnant, and that outcome brought us together. We were supposed to get married and we did. Do you know how good it feels to finally accept this? Do you know how easy it is for me to deal with what happened because it was supposed to be? I'm glad I got pregnant and I'm glad we got married. "Why not, Jeff?"

The second *why me* question that has tormented me for years was *why did you stay married to me*? Can you imagine how painful this *why me* issue was? You were a bisexual man who wanted a gay lifestyle. *Why did you remain with me all these years when you were sexually attracted to men*? I know we had a lot of things in common and we were best friends. We cared deeply about each other and we were a great team. We had fun, shared ideas, goals, and interests. We complemented each other. But, you were having sexual relations with other men. *Why did you want me?* What disturbed me even more was *why did I stay with you? Why couldn't we walk away from each other and the marriage? Why Jeff?* I asked myself these questions twenty-four hours a day, seven days a week. It consumed me. How many arguments did we have about this? How many times did I scream at you, *"why do you stay with me and why can't you leave?"* The more I asked you these questions, the more my anger towards you grew. Saying *"why me"* hurt so badly, I wanted to hurt you back.

Again, how I looked at this issue made all the difference. When I changed the *why me* to the *why not me,* the anger and resentment towards you left. When I said, *why not me* I felt good about us and was glad we'd fought to keep our marriage together. Saying *why not me* made everything easy and natural. Adding the word *not* gave me something I'd never known before. Peace of mind. So now I say, *"Why shouldn't we have stayed together and tried to make our marriage work?"* All married couples have their problems. We continued to work on our relationship and focus on the wonderful things we shared. We had fun, laughed and talked about everything. We wanted each other to succeed and were never threatened by the other one's accomplishments. We cared and respected each other, as friends should. We stayed together because *this was the kind of relationship we were supposed to have.* Accepting that enabled me to find my inner self and let go once and for all of the pain.

The third *why me* question was the most disturbing one of all. It caused me to hate my own existence and almost cost me my life. The question was *why did AIDS happen? Why did this horrible illness come along?*

Why did you have to get this disease? Why did you do this to yourself and why did you do this to me? You took your beautiful body, a wonderful life, and destroyed it because of sex. I hated you for getting ill and ruining our lives. And I'm going to hate you for dying and leaving me alone. All I wanted was for you to be here with me sharing our life and future together. Facing these *why* questions caused me the most pain and anguish I'd ever known. They made me want to die, because I knew I'd still be alive after you were gone.

How did I get rid of this *why me* pain and anger that almost drove me to kill myself? The *why me* had to become the *why not me*. AIDS wasn't a curse, a plaque, or a wrath from God. Men in white coats working in laboratories didn't invent this virus to kill *gay men*. It wasn't exclusive to drug addicts or prostitutes. It wasn't a disease sent down to earth as punishment for people's sins. AIDS is a disease. Like many others before it, this disease causes great pain and suffering. Unfortunately, like many others, it is fatal. Innocent people will get life-threatening diseases and die. Life isn't fair and no one is exempt from it. Death is an unavoidable part of life. The *why me person* couldn't exist anymore. I wouldn't have been able to write my feelings down and I wouldn't have been able to tell others. The *why not me* person is dealing with these questions and handling them. The *why not me* woman is getting stronger and feels more in control. Saying *"why not me"* has given me the courage to face my fears. I know that my life has turned out the way it was supposed to. As a *why not me* person, I'll make my own decisions and accept their consequences. I don't want to know *why* any longer and I'll never let a *why me* question affect my life or cloud my judgment again.

Along my journey, I'll have to handle many more difficult situations. Some of these experiences will only challenge me while others will alter the course of my life. My darling, I've finally come to terms with the three hardest questions I've wrestled with for twenty-three years. Why did I get pregnant? Why did you stay with me? Why did you get AIDS and die? I had to learn how to deal with these powerful issues in a way that was positive or their destructive forces would have taken my life. It took me a long time to understand that, probably because I really didn't want to. My healing process began when I started to deal openly and honestly with my problems. "Life doesn't have to make sense to make sense." Having a reason and purpose is good enough. I know, in the future, I'm capable of becoming a happier person. I accept the fact that I'm totally responsible for my actions, choices, and conduct. No one can force or threaten me to do anything I don't want to do. They can try, but the *why not me* person won't let them succeed. I'll have many options in the future and I'll make the decisions I'm supposed to make. Nothing in my life has been a mistake and every decision I've made has been the right one. We both made sacrifices and compromised many times to stay in our passionate and tumultuous marriage, but "WHY NOT?" We were supposed to and the *why not me* would do it all over again.

Saturday, June 27, 1992

Dear Jeff,

Where has the past week gone? As I sit next to your bed today watching you sleep, I know my prayers have been answered. You have come through this initial crisis and you are going to live. I knew if anyone could have pulled through this, you could. You had the finest doctors and medical care available. You also had an endless supply of love and support from your family and friends. But, I personally felt that something much more powerful was helping you during this time. I honestly and unconditionally believed that your life was now in God's hands. Since there wasn't anything else anyone could do for you, I resigned myself to the fact that if you recovered it was because God wanted it that way. As I've done in the past, I put all my faith and confidence into my spiritual beliefs. I had to trust in God and that faith gave me the strength, peace, and comfort I desperately needed now. If I hadn't done that, I would have failed us both. I know without any hesitation that a much higher power has guided and watched over us through this terrible time. Though I've been challenged and frightened many times during the past week, I felt that my God was with me and I didn't feel alone.

You know how difficult the religious aspect of my life has been for me to accept. I have always felt spiritually close to my own personal God, but I haven't been consistently faithful in my beliefs. This past year has tested my faith more than any other time in my life. As I've watched this disease slowly take over your body, my religious convictions have been seriously challenged. I've been confronted with questions and issues I've never wanted to address before. I have been afraid to open myself up to feelings so intensely personal and private that I've never been able to talk about them to anyone. I never even shared my thoughts with you. Until this very moment, I wasn't sure what I could handle, what I believed in, or if I could believe at all. Only through my writing am I able to ask myself, "Is this what the past year has been for? Is your illness the reason why I must finally deal with my fears and doubts concerning my spiritual beliefs? Has the time come for me to ask myself once and for all, do I really believe in God? Has your illness also forced me to take an honest look at my own mortality? This is an issue that has always been too frightening for me to personally address."

As I look back over my childhood years, I know that I didn't like the hypocrisy I saw in my strict Orthodox Jewish upbringing. The old-fashioned Judaic principles and kosher rules my family adhered to caused me much confusion and doubt. This wasn't the way I wanted to carry out my religious ideals. My faith came from my heart, not from useless practices I found unnecessary. My God would know me by what I did for others, not for what others thought I should do. And so over the years, I've challenged my beliefs many times during our marriage. I haven't understood why I've always needed a sign or some evidence that God existed. How often did I say to you, "Jeff, I envy those who truly believe in God?" Why can't I have that unwavering acceptance of a divine presence in my life? Why don't I have that undoubting faith I know others possessed? Did I use my faith as a crutch, only believing when times were difficult or when everything seemed hopeless? Were my words paying lip service to help me through my darkest hours? Was I a hypocrite because I asked for

God's help only when faced with adversity or hardship? When my life was running smoothly and the times were good, why did I need to believe in God? Did I ask for God's help but fail to give thanks when I received what I had asked for? These questions have haunted me during this past year and now as I write I will face my fears once and for all.

A few weeks ago I was at the lowest point in my life. I felt helpless, hopeless, and disheartened. I almost packed my suitcases and ran away. I wanted to be rid of you, my life, and my pain. I went out on the balcony and as I watched a million stars brilliantly shining above me I screamed, "God, why have you made my life so difficult and presented me with these challenges? Why have you given me so many burdens to carry around? I don't understand why life should be so terribly cruel. Why would you want anyone to go through this kind of torment and suffering? Why, God, are you doing this terrible thing to us? Why does this wonderful man have AIDS?" Just writing this down causes my hands to shake and my body to tremble. Part of me understands that I will not make it through this time without God's help. But, how do I allow myself to unconditionally believe? How can I put all my faith and trust into something I have never been certain about? If I have doubted my faith in the past, how can I be sure that I will never doubt again? And, if I doubt my God now, where will I find the strength in the future? My heart is broken and I don't know what to do. Once and for all I must either accept God's presence in my life or I must stop pretending. During the past week, I realized that praying and believing were the only things alleviating my doubts and fears. In these, my darkest hours, my faith in God is all I have. I hope I will not disappoint my God or disappoint myself even more.

Since I am certain now that you will recover, I have made my final decision. I have accepted God's presence in my life and I will never doubt that faith again. I know why I have been constantly tested throughout our marriage. I was supposed to go through these hardships and troubled times because I had to find out that my God was within me. To finally accept God into my life, I had to give myself permission to let that feeling in. It has been through my doubts and fears that I have reached this higher level of understanding about myself. If I ask the same questions I did before with an open mind and a believing heart, I will find the strength I need to carry on. If I couldn't resolve my problems before, it was because I didn't know where to find the solutions. If I have suffered alone for too long in the past, I do not want to suffer any longer. If I have been tormented for years because I questioned the power of my beliefs, I do not want to torment myself any more. If I have felt alone and helpless, it was because I wouldn't allow my God to take my sorrow away. I was a stranger to myself because I doubted my faith. Now, I have the peace of mind I desperately need because I have turned my anger and sorrow over to my God. If I didn't want to believe before you took ill, it is the only thing I want to do now.

Also during the past week, I have reached a plateau with your condition. I have made a gradual transition from anger, to denial, to final acceptance. I've actually adjusted to the insanity around me. I am getting comfortable with the day's routine and I am feeling some stability. I almost know what to expect and I have gotten accustomed to certain things. I do not feel as panicked or fearful at this time. I am feeling more in control of my emotions and feelings as I accept what is going on around me. I know you will get well and that you will go home. That is why today I can honestly address the acceptance of God's presence in my life. There had to be a reason why you were supposed to live. Maybe I don't know at this moment what all those reasons are, but God has a plan for me, for us, and for AIDS. How can I doubt this? Instead of this disease destroying us, we will face it together and it will keep us together. Does God want you to live because we have other matters to complete? Was I supposed to doubt my faith and be tested by this disease? Yes, Jeff, because once I made the decision to believe, it became my only weapon against an unbeatable foe. If we were to face your long and difficult recovery together, I would never be able to doubt my God again.

While I was praying for your recovery, I was searching for my own personal relationship with God. And what time could challenge me more than a life-threatening illness like AIDS? Would there ever be another period in my life that would cause me such doubt and fear? Recognizing this fact and having doubts about my beliefs was exactly what I was supposed to do. Questioning the presence of that higher being and doubting the existence of a spiritual power was the only way I could finally accept this feeling. I have gained strength by facing this ordeal and have come to terms with the power of my convictions. I am thankful for your spared life and the time we have together. If I have always believed that I was on a journey through life, then this was a part of it. The more I've searched to find out what I do believe in, the less I've been able to find out. The more I've questioned my faith and challenged my beliefs, the more I realize that I am dealing with them. By allowing myself to feel vulnerable and doubtful, I have gained confidence and strength. If I have to confront other difficult issues in the future, I know I will face them with hope, faith, and my God's support.

8 The Frustration Factor

"The only thing stable about my life is the instability."

Tuesday, June 23, 1992

Dear Jeff,

The doctor said your condition is guarded but he was optimistic about your latest test results. I don't think the reality of this has fully set in because I'm still in a state of shock after hearing your diagnosis with pneumonia and AIDS. I thought I was prepared for the worst, but now I know I was not. I feel like I am in a trance or some hypnotic state, performing out of habit just going through the motions. I am functioning and existing in a perpetual state of gray in an endless fog that will not lift. Nothing is clear and I feel my world has collapsed around me. My mind is going in every direction at once. I am confused, terrified, and feel emotionally out of control. I am overwhelmed with feelings so intense and extreme that I do not know which ones I can deal with first. I am not able to focus on anything and my writing is the one thing bringing me comfort and peace. It has been the only manageable way for me to sort out my feelings. Through my writing, I will remember all the details I wished I could forget. Doesn't that sound insane? I want to forget everything but I know I must not. The only way I will get through this time is to let my words express my feelings. I don't know where to begin and I'm not even sure if my writing will make any sense.

This was the first time I had ever faced a medical crisis and how much worse could it have been? You had a life-threatening illness and a deadly bacterial infection. When you were diagnosed last Friday, all I could think about was getting you to the hospital safely the following morning. Once I got you there, I didn't even know if you would survive. Would your condition stabilize? When would they let me see you? Would they let me stay in the room with you overnight? My poor darling, you were so afraid. I wanted you to know that I would never leave you alone. Then there were all the forms and paperwork to take care of. I don't remember signing those. I don't recall to whom I spoke, or how long it took to get you into a room. I thought about the hospital. Though, I knew you were receiving excellent medical attention, would it be the best? There were so many new doctors and nurses, it took all my energy and concentration just to remember their names. And what about the drugs and treatments you had to receive? I didn't know anything about the AIDS drugs they would give you to treat the pneumonia. The doctors couldn't give me any guarantees that any of them worked. And what do I tell the other family members and our close friends? How much information should I give them? How long would you be here? Would you be transferred to another hospital? Everything was so overwhelming. The big decisions were monumental and the little ones were enormous. The only thing stable about my life at this moment was the instability.

It is 1992 and AIDS is still a relatively unknown disease. People are fearful and taking every precaution guarding against the possibility of HIV transmission. The facts and data about the drugs are not specific, and the specialty of infectious diseases is unknown to me. Though I have complete trust and faith in our doctor, I do not know any of the others specialists who will be involved with your treatment. Our hospital is modern and well equipped, but is it the right one for your illness? This issue has been tormenting me for days. On one hand, I want them to do whatever they have to do to keep you alive. On the other hand, I question every test, drug, and procedure they are performing. You have suffered so much already and I don't want them to cause you any more pain. I have to believe that everyone is doing the best they can and that I have made the right decisions about your care. Your parents were equally afraid, yet, they trust my judgement. They need my reassurance that everything will be all right. How can I reassure them when I have so many doubts and concerns myself?

I sit here writing watching as your life rests in everyone else's hands. People are coming in and out of your room constantly taking blood, checking your vital signs, changing out IV bags, and reading the monitors. They are waking you up at all hours of the day and night asking you questions you can't understand. I feel like a team of robots has invaded our life. Each one precisely performing their delegated duties and assigned tasks. Though I know they are trying to save your life, they are a constant source of agitation and disruption. As I lay next to you on a cot, in a cold, dark, sterile, hospital room, the antiseptic stench burns my nostrils. With every shift change comes a new staff of nurses, aids, and lab technicians. I want them to give you more personal attention so I try to tell them about you, what you'd been through and how wonderful you are. I want them to know you as I do and I desperately want them to know how much I love you. I want them to treat you like they would their family. I try to be tactful and considerate of them because I want them to like you. I am frightened, but I try to be considerate and polite to them. But, sometimes panic and fear takes over and I become rude, angry, and demanding. I fear they will get upset with me and they might overlook some small detail because of something I said or did. That sounds like something a paranoid person would say, but this is how I feel.

The two most powerful feelings I am experiencing now are shock and terror. I call this state I'm in "my fear factor", because the fear of not knowing what might happen during the next few days is unbearable. I am my own worst enemy. I am a prisoner being held captive by my thoughts. My world has been turned upside down and I am in turmoil. My life has no purpose any longer and I can't find a safe place within myself "to just be." I feel I am dangerously close to an emotional collapse. I watch, wait, and hope that you will survive. The only thing I want is for you to live. I cannot make decisions or plans about tomorrow because I do not know if there will be a tomorrow with you. I ask myself over and over again why did this happen? What will I do next? How will I go on? And, finally, the most dreaded one of all. Are you going to die? My questions cannot be answered and this uncertainty has me paralyzed. The more I try to convince myself to step back and let go, the more I want to crawl into a corner and hide. I don't know if or how I will be able to handle anything again.

Maybe the best way to express the way I feel is, it's manageable chaos. Everything around me is out of control, but there is an organized plan to this madness. It reminds me of a stage production with the same show appearing every day, every night, 365 days a year. As I write these thoughts down I'm actually smiling because in some bizarre way, this scenario makes sense to me. I shall call my play, "The Frustration Factor." The hospital and rooms are the setting for this production. The medical staff are the producers, directors, and stagehands while the patients are the actors and actresses. There are never any dress rehearsals or understudies. Sometimes, the performances are perfect and the show goes off without a hitch. The applause is for a job well done and everyone is pleased with the reviews. But sometimes, there are missed cues, forgotten lines, and the show is terrible. When this happens the actor/patient pays the price, takes the blame, and suffers the consequences. I had a front row seat to a show I didn't want to see and when the curtain came down, all I wanted was for us to go home.

My darling, I didn't believe in miracles before, but I do now. Something just happened to me that I can't explain. As I was writing, I started to feel better. I was able to sort out my thoughts and was able to regain some order and focus back into my life. I think the shock phase of this time had finally left me and I was feeling hopeful. It's like I'd taken my first deep breath of fresh air in days and it felt wonderful. I thought we just might make it through this after all. I was more comfortable with myself and was beginning to feel alive again. I knew in my heart that nothing had changed concerning your illness, but I knew I was handling my emotions better. The surprising thing was that it happened so quickly and it happened to both of us. One moment you were sleeping and the next minute you were looking at me asking what I was writing about. You smiled, took the pen from my hand, and said, "You've been a busy lady, haven't you?" You began asking me questions about your illness, how long you had been here, and what your doctors were doing. You were finally responding to the treatments and we were both getting better together. You asked me to call your parents and have them bring over a hamburger, French fries, and a chocolate shake. You were speaking clearly, your voice was stronger, and you wanted something to eat. I knew then that we would make it through your recovery together. Thanks for coming back to me. I need you.

9 *Personal Touches in an Impersonal Environment*

June 29, 1992

Dear Jeff,

You went into the hospital to get better, but even as sick as you were, you hated every minute of it. You've never liked going to the doctor, or waiting for an appointment, and you were a very difficult patient. When we went to get our marriage license and the nurse took your blood, you fainted. It took her ten minutes to revive you. A few months after we got married, I begged you to let me clean your teeth. You came to the VA Hospital and no sooner had I begun did you grab the instruments from my hands, flew out of the chair, and drove home. You didn't speak to me about it for two days. You choked on pills, threw up when medications didn't taste good, and thought that the hospital was a place where people checked in and didn't always come out. And you certainly would have starved to death if it meant eating institutional food. If you had your way, the hospital would have been set up in our home. But, you didn't have any choice. Your worst case scenario had come true and nobody could tell us how long it would continue.

For the first few days, you were oblivious to everything around you. I was very protective and concerned about your safety and well-being and it was my responsibility to make sure you got whatever you required. I went home only to freshen up and bring you back something you might need. I asked for a special recliner chair/bed to be put in the room so that I could spend the nights with you. I wanted to be close by to call for help if something unforeseen happened. Since your condition was critical, the staff was very thankful I was staying in the room. Night after night, you woke around 2:00 AM delirious with fever, anxious, and frightened. Your recovery was going to be agonizingly slow and overwhelmingly frustrating. Some days your progress was visibly apparent, while other times your setbacks only reinforced how ill you really were. I found myself writing at all hours of the day and night. I documented the procedures, your treatments and medications, and recorded the names of everyone who came into your room. The more information I detailed and outlined in my journals, the more valuable they became as a resource and reference guide for your illness and recovery.

I loathed the constant confusion and disturbances during the first few days. Everything was in turmoil and nothing seemed to be going right. I referred to this time as my energy drains because all of my energy was going out and nothing was coming in. I realized that the issues of privacy, self-respect, and your pride became very important. Since your appearance always meant so much to you, it was heart breaking and embarrassing for you to have people see you this way. Between the medical staff, your immediate family, and a few close friends, people were constantly coming in and out of the room. We didn't have any privacy and I missed our "alone times" together. I tried to screen the phone calls, but it was very difficult to refuse anyone's best wishes and prayers. People wanted to let us know how much they cared. Whenever someone did visit, I'd find myself crying because I felt their sadness when they saw how ill you were. That was another reason why my writing became so important to me. If we couldn't be alone, I knew I could share my private thoughts and feelings with you on paper.

You always trusted my judgement and common sense, but now there was so much pressure and responsibility on me. I didn't know what decisions were right or wrong. When could you have visitors? Who could visit and for how long? If someone offered to bring something, what was appropriate? I didn't know what to expect and I couldn't make any plans because you might be having a treatment, or be violently ill, or sleeping. Since there were so many procedures constantly being done to you, how much energy did you have left for company? Everyone wanted to be involved and meant only the best, but if you were to regain your strength, I had to be very firm and specific about these things. Until the day came that you were strong enough to make these decisions again, I had to determine what was best for you.

Besides writing, I knew I had to have something productive and physical to do. You were terrified about everything and this cold bleak hospital room only added to your misery. How could I stand by and allow you to be in this place day after day and not try to make you feel better? I realized that if I was to have any impact on your recovery, I could try and make your hospital stay more comfortable. I believed that your mental and emotional attitude would improve more quickly if the room felt more like home. Since you might have to be here for several weeks, I wanted you to feel a sense of belonging to the life you left and hopefully would return to. What could I do to make your room feel more homey and cheerful? I could bring your personal things and our home to you. I endeavored to make this unfamiliar place look familiar. I wanted to fill your room with life, energy, and give it a healthy new look with hope.

I made a list of the little things that I could bring to you. I wanted you to be surrounded with things that were peaceful and soothing. I brought in several large pictures from our vacations and a few special pieces of artwork. You especially loved the picture of us standing on the cliff at Moraine Lake in British Columbia, Canada. It was the most tranquil setting and the breathtaking watercolors always made you happy and smile. I put it on the window ledge where you stared at it for hours. I filled a suitcase up with souvenirs, clothes, colognes, and other personal items. I found our Beetle records and we listened to disco music from the 70's and 80's on my boom box stereo. I put our high school and college yearbooks in a large brown tote bag and brought them over at 3:00

AM. We laughed about the clothes and our "in" looks over the years. When people asked what they could bring on their visits, I said anything festive, full of life, and fun. Within the week, we had a room full of balloons, flowers, and chocolates.

The next thing I had to deal with was how to get you to eat. I watched you getting weaker and weaker during the past six months. You had lost a considerable amount of weight. Our mealtimes had become terribly tense and brought much conflict and hostility between us. Your immune system was seriously compromised, your appetite diminished, and now you were too sick to care. You couldn't take solid foods and liquids were given to you in IV solutions. When your meals were brought in you might be coughing so violently that you couldn't catch your breath. In between the 104 degree fevers and the convulsions, you had dry heaves. For several days, I watched helplessly as your meal trays went untouched. It was a futile, frustrating, and distressing issue for us to deal with. The medicines could combat the bacterial infection, but you needed to eat if you were going to regain your strength. My battle cry became, "Please eat and drink, Jeff. Just do something. How can you fight this disease and get well when you won't eat?" But, nothing I said or did worked.

To compound everything else, you hated the hospital food. You threw up several times just looking at the trays. Food had always been an important part of our marriage and since you loved my cooking I brought the finest and healthiest food to you. This was equally important for me because it gave my life purpose and meaning again. You were in a private room so I brought in an ice chest, a small refrigerator, and our own microwave. If you wanted something, I rushed home, made it, and brought it back. For two weeks, you had home-cooked lunches and dinners brought in daily. I even served you on china, with silverware. We did use hospital linens for napkins. I stocked the ice chest with cold drinks, juices, and filled the room with assorted snacks, crackers, candy bars, chips, and anything extra that you might want. Your restaurant was brought to you. And slowly but steadily you started to respond. Your appetite was coming back and you were eating. Our doctor said that my meals were "IBMs" or itsy bitsy miracles. I had developed a routine of cooking, serving, and delivering that would continue as long as you were here. The only goal I had in mind was to fatten you up, get you stronger, and bring you home.

There was one other thing I could do for you that might speed up your recovery. I had to show you that I was taking care of myself. I was no good to you or your parents if I didn't get my act together. You needed me more than ever and seeing me look the way I did was the worst thing I could be doing for you. I remember the day you looked at me and said, "Susan, I'm the one who is sick. Please look like the woman I need back in my life." That was my wake up call. You deserved the wife you had always known and I wouldn't fail you. From now on, when you saw me come into your room, I looked like the lady you always admired and loved. I put on your favorite perfume, wore something pretty and bright, and looked like I was going to make it through this time too. I was emotionally and physically exhausted, but I looked and acted like the woman you needed back. You had many things to live for and I was one of them.

And so my darling, you gave me a challenge during those two weeks, but I think your hospital room looked pretty damn good. This room was our home for a while but you were surrounded with people who loved you, delicious home cooked meals, festive decorations, and hope. That was the one thing I truly wanted to give you. I tried to keep things as comfortable as possible here and at home. Whenever you returned to our house, it would look just as beautiful as you remembered. We were going to make it together.

Friday, July 3, 1992

Dear Jeff,

I am both apprehensive and excited at the same time. I feel like I am bringing a baby home instead of my husband. It is a catch-22. The hospital gave me a sense of security because you were safe and you were being taken care of there. Though I desperately wanted you home, I have mixed emotions about today. I've planned ahead for your homecoming because I wanted you to feel comfortable and relaxed when you came back from the hospital. Prioritizing everything regarding your comfort and well-being are my major concerns. I feel compassion for what you have been through and I want to be as considerate of your needs as possible. I am writing everything down in detail and will be "rigidly flexible" in sticking to my lists. I've gone through the house and gathered up all your previous medications and supplies. I dated, named, and sealed them in individual zip lock bags. Since I didn't want you to see these items when you came home, I placed them away in the closet in a large see through plastic blanket box. The compressor for your daily inhalation treatments was delivered and put in the laundry room. Your refrigerated medications are dated and stored in a separate bin away from the food. I brought your personal belongings home from the hospital first. Then, I went back and signed the discharge papers, filled your prescriptions, obtained the doctors' phone numbers, and finally picked you up. It is a holiday weekend and there aren't many people at the hospital. I need to be prepared for any emergency or crisis that could arise.

It was extremely hot when I dropped you off at the apartment. I feared the short walk to the elevator would tire you out. I'd always been overly protective and the title Mother Hen certainly applied now. However, my fears vanished when I saw the look on your face as we walked through the door of our apartment together. You said, "Bee, it's the most beautiful home in the world. Thank you for loving me." The artwork, pictures, and other treasured pieces from our travels were just as you remembered. A large balloon bouquet with a welcome home banner hung from the ceiling fan. Fresh flowers were everywhere and the house was filled with life, love, and happiness. Dozens of cards were strung across the room. The refrigerator and pantry were stocked with your favorite foods. I couldn't believe that on Friday, July 3, at 6:00 PM, you were sleeping in our bed. It looked like nothing ever happened and you were on the road to recovery.

You woke up groggy and disoriented, but when you came into the kitchen and asked, "What's for dinner?" I started to cry. I said, "Cheeseburgers and candy bars made with real meat and chocolate." We couldn't stop laughing because we were both so health conscious and now I was thinking "fat." I put two giant cheeseburgers, a baked potato with sour cream and butter, a salad with Russian dressing, and a Milky Way candy bar on your plate. I wanted this meal to be fun and special. You ate the Milky Way first. It was wonderful watching you do it. You looked at me and said, "I think eating again will be fun." I said, "You'll love putting those twenty pounds back on again." However, that was more difficult to do than we imagined. Sometimes you wanted to eat, then without notice you lost your appetite. Some medications had to be taken on an empty stomach, while others required food. In between your coughing

SUSAN MINTZ | 98

spells, nausea, and diarrhea, it was difficult for you to gain and maintain your weight.

The three things you needed most were to eat, rest, and relax. Everything we did for the next few weeks revolved around those issues. Establishing a routine was not easy because there were many people involved with your care. Between your daily inhalation treatments, regularly scheduled visits from home health personnel, laboratory pick-ups, and equipment and medication deliveries, we were always waiting for someone to arrive or something to be dropped off. If we were going to get our life back together, it was up to me to coordinate the appointments and familiarize myself with these matters. The phone situation was the first problem I had to deal with. Because you weren't sleeping well at night, you tired easily and were taking frequent naps during the day. The phone calls were constant and becoming annoying and disturbing. It was different when you first took ill. I welcomed the support from family and friends and their kindness and concern for us was exactly what I needed during those first two weeks. But, now the constant phone calls were waking you up, interrupting your treatments, and disturbing our meals. They were intruding on our private time together and disrupting your recovery. I was very adamant about the telephone situation and stressed what I felt was best for you.

We decided for the first few days until we got organized, I would tell family and friends that when you were sleeping I was taking the phone off the hook. If you had the energy after you woke up and wanted to speak with someone that was up to you. If not, I would handle the phone calls myself. I had to be honest with everyone and stated that you needed this time to regain your strength. I couldn't be more specific because we were trying to get a routine established and our life back on track. I told your parents that I would call them twice a day and keep them informed about everything that was going on. They were the only ones who had "carte blanche" to their son and when you wanted them to visit, I picked them up. For several weeks, in order to maintain our privacy and conserve your energy, I felt it was my responsibility to handle the telephone situation. Eventually, you would have plenty of time for visitors and phone calls.

Since you were very weak and didn't have the energy to go out, I decided to bring the entertainment to you. We loved going to the movies. Remember how many times we did three shows in one day? We called them our "marathon watches." We had so many to get caught up on and it was something we looked forward to. Every day, I picked a movie that seemed appropriate for our dinner. At 8:00 PM, I rang the dinner bell. We went into the den, and I served you the "specialty of the house." For several weeks, we had front row seats to the best show in town. I'd watch you eat, relax, and fall asleep during it. I was so excited the first night you ate your entire dinner and stayed awake through the entire movie that I got the camera out and took a picture of your empty plate.

I eventually had to address the issue concerning our sleeping arrangements. You used to say, "we were playing spoons" because we fit so well when we slept together. I cherished the nights when you held me in your arms. You always me feel safe and secure. I thought since the pneumonia was gone we would be able to sleep together again. But, your sleeping habits had changed and it was difficult being in the same bed with you. You were restless, ran low-grade fevers, had night sweats, coughed, and snored. You always complained that your legs were jumpy and you couldn't find a place for yourself. I put nightlights around the room because when you woke up you were groggy and bumped into things. There was a pitcher of ice water near the bed at all times because you woke up thirsty several times during the night. Sleeping together was once easy, comfortable, and natural, but now it had become a difficult and uncomfortable nightly situation. Getting into bed caused us great tension and my agitation caused me to lose patience with you. Rather than cause you any further stress, I chose to sleep in another bedroom. If we were to adjust to our new life together, our communication would have to be better than ever.

Every morning for the next few weeks, we made tentative plans for the day and thought about what we might want to do. You were getting stronger, staying awake longer, tolerating your inhalation treatments, and feeling better. We started to have visitors in and you began taking short walks. Your appetite was definitely coming back and you put on three pounds the first week. You were so excited and came flying out of the bathroom that morning. We celebrated with cake and ice cream for breakfast. As long as I focused on your best interests, I knew I could get you well again. We used our time effectively. It didn't matter how long it took for you to recover. We were settling into a lifestyle and routine that took a lot of time, organization, and prioritizing, but it was paying off.

By the end of September, you were really feeling better. We had become familiar, knowledgeable, and confident with every aspect of this disease. We learned to understand the physical, psychological, and emotional issues we faced. By working together, we managed to become stable and comfortable with our situation. We accepted the disease as a part of our life, worked around it, and tried not to control it. But organization was the key word. I continued to document everything in my journals keeping precise records of your temperatures, side effects from the medications, or any other symptoms you might develop. The more detailed I was, the more information I had to give the doctors and data I had to compare it with. The doctors didn't have a specific plan of attack and they weren't sure what all the options were. A lot of your recovery was based on how well your body responded to the treatments. Regaining your appetite, energy, and maintaining a healthy lifestyle helped in your remarkable recovery over the next three months.

I look back on that Saturday morning, July 4th, when you came out of the bedroom and said, "What's for breakfast?" Everything we ever were or were to be was tested when you became ill. But tonight, we held each other under a starlit magical sky and celebrated life, love, and your recovery. We watched fireworks exploding around us and the balmy night air caressed our skin. Nothing terrible happened to us tonight and this perfect evening shall remain in my memory forever. I never want to say good-bye to you again. I loved you more tonight than ever before and that strength and devotion will help you heal.

11 Baby Steps

October 1, 1992

Dear Jeff,

The long and challenging summer of '92 has come and gone. Do you remember watching the movie, "Baby Steps?" In this comedy, Richard Dreyfuss plays a psychiatrist treating Bill Murray who has suffered for years with numerous fears and phobias. Throughout the movie the term baby steps came to signify the slow continuous progress that was accomplished even though the progress wasn't always apparent. For me, now, the words baby steps have become both personal and painful, because they represent some of the most difficult and frustrating times we experienced as you recovered from pneumonia.

I watched this disease ravish your physical, mental, and emotional well-being. Our challenges were made more difficult and complicated because we didn't know what to expect or how much progress you would make. If you were to recover, we had to honestly believe that you could never stop taking your "baby steps." You took some steps forwards, some backwards, but most of them felt as if you weren't going anywhere. We were frustrated and fearful, but our goal was to continue working our way back to a quality of life we would enjoy again. Taking "baby steps", one day at a time, kept us positive and was our therapy helping you to get well. "Baby Steps" became my mantra and continued keeping me focused on a very uncertain future.

This was phase one of your recovery process. We were starting over and everything we did became a first. My one priority was helping you to get your appetite back. You couldn't regain your strength if you wouldn't eat. I diligently planned our meals hoping that something appealed to you, but for days I watched as you picked at your food. You couldn't chew and breathe at the same time because you were constantly coughing. It was obvious that you were forcing yourself to eat. Then, one evening you actually finished your entire dinner. It took six weeks for that first to happen. It was a celebration of accomplishment and determination. Twelve weeks after your diagnosis, we realized your cough had finally stopped, you weren't nauseous, and didn't have diarrhea during or after dinner.

Three months of frustration and sometimes desperation trying to get you to eat was finally paying off. I somehow managed to work my little "baby step miracles" in the kitchen and you were regaining your health as well as your confidence. One night you wanted to go out for dinner and said, "I want a double cheese, pepperoni, garlic, and anchovy pizza." I said, "You don't like anchovies." You said, "I'll eat anything now." You started going to the market and picking out what you wanted to eat. I pushed you out the door yelling, "Please go and buy out the entire store." Your improvement was so gradual that sometimes it wasn't obvious. And my greatest pleasure was when you woke up in the middle of the night and said you were hungry. I was so happy I couldn't stop crying. I never thought I would hear those words again. By the end of September, you'd gained back the twenty pounds you lost in the hospital. Those three months went from "baby steps" to a "giant step" and it was well worth the wait.

For twenty-three years, you were the most wonderful man to sleep with. You didn't snore, never woke up during the night, and in the morning you wanted to take on the world. How could anyone have so much energy and enthusiasm that early in the day? As your pneumonia worsened, so did your sleeping habits. You hadn't had a restful night's sleep in months. When you came home from the hospital, all you did for weeks was sleep and nap during the day. You could barely stay awake during dinner and couldn't watch TV for more than an hour without falling asleep. Eating and talking on the telephone exhausted you. You were still spiking fevers and breaking out in drenching night sweats. You woke several times during the night extremely thirsty, wanting something to drink. You needed help getting to the bathroom because you were weak and disoriented.

Weeks went by when one day you said, "I don't need to lie down. I'm going to my desk and pay the bills." I said, "You hate paying the bills." You said, "I'm so happy to have the energy to do it." For weeks, you couldn't keep your eyes open during a movie. Then, one afternoon you wanted to go to the theater. It was the first time in months we watched the end of a movie together. One morning we woke up and realized you hadn't had a night sweat in days. We went to bed that evening laughing about the "soup kitchen" I was running. Your improvement was slowly happening. You were sleeping better, eating more, and feeling optimistic about the future. It took three long and difficult months making those "baby steps" work. But our "firsts" felt wonderful.

You were always a physical person lifting weights, riding a bicycle, dancing, swimming, and walking. The pneumonia weakened you terribly and the lack of physical activity caused your muscles to atrophy. When you came home from the hospital, you couldn't walk to the bathroom alone. Your legs were wobbly and you were dizzy. I followed you around for days because I was fearful you might fall. You would have to push yourself in order to regain your strength. Starting an exercise program again posed many difficult, demanding, and painful challenges. Several times a day, you walked around the apartment. Each time, you walked a little longer and you felt stronger. One day, I called to you but you didn't answer. I was terrified that you had fallen down. The door opened and you had the mail in your hands. I yelled at you for scaring me, but I was so excited because you felt strong enough to go downstairs and get the mail.

I remember the first time we took a walk around the block and the sprinklers went off. You ran through them with a burst of energy I hadn't seen in weeks. The first time you rode the stationary bike again for ten minutes you thought you would faint. But every day, you rode the bike, increasing your time a little more. One day you rode forty minutes and you weren't even breathing hard. I remember the first time you wanted to drive the car. We went dancing under a moonlit sky holding each other to the song "Hold Me." After three months you had your strength and energy back again. We were walking on the beach, enjoying all the activities we used to do. Your progress was so subtle and gradual that sometimes we didn't notice it, but those physical "baby steps" eventually paid off.

Your emotional "baby steps" were the hardest to deal with. The stress had us on a roller coaster ride from hell. Regaining our emotional stability required tremendous patience, love, and determination twenty-four hours a day. We experienced fear, anger, resentment, depression and periods of isolation. You were frustrated and frightened. You suffered from anxiety attacks. These feelings and emotions were unpredictable, powerful, and as harmful as the deadly virus you carried. You had to find a way to cope with your fears as you learned to live with this disease. The issues were compounded because AIDS didn't have any cure and your prognosis wasn't good. There were many unknown factors involved and you were apprehensive about the treatments and medications. Your doctors were bombarding you with facts, figures and clinical data that disturbed and confused you even more. You had difficulty just getting up the courage to look at your lab results. You became depressed because your blood work never came back "normal" and your counts were all out of range. It was a long and tedious process, but you began working around the disease. You established a new lifestyle and routine as you took your emotional "baby steps." You accepted your illness and started to take back control of your life.

We also had to learn how to laugh and have fun again. It was hard to feel happy when everything around us was so sad. The weeks went by and we talked more, shared our thoughts, and rationalized our situation. But, we couldn't find anything to make us feel good again. I remember the first time we actually laughed. You came home from having a chest x-ray at the hospital. You had a 100-degree fever and were freezing. You wanted to try and eat something, so we sat down for dinner. You were playing with a meatball and twirling the spaghetti around in circles when you broke out in a drenching sweat. You started to laugh and said, "I think it's something in the sauce that broke my fever." We spent so much time talking about eating, why not make food the brunt of our jokes? That's when we started to laugh and have fun. We got hysterical as I made my famous concoctions in an attempt to get you to take your medications. You especially liked the pills in the Snickers Bar dessert. You went to the refrigerator and took out the real butter, sour cream, mayonnaise, and said this getting well diet wasn't so terrible.

Another difficult issue was your wetting the bed problem. You broke out in horrible night sweats that drenched the sheets. You moved over to my side of the bed. I'd place several bath towels over the wet area, and I'd lie on top of them. There were times, however, when at 3:00 AM, we were changing the sheets. One night you yelled, "let's invest in a laundromat or use disposable sheets and linens." We started making fun of our nightly event and it became part of the wellness comedy club routine. You also liked when I dressed up and played the exterminator during your weekly inhalation treatments. I would glove up, put on a mask, and hook you up to the compressor. You had to walk around for twenty minutes breathing from a long plastic tube that came out of a huge blue mouthpiece. We looked like something out of a sci-fi movie. These scenes weren't funny, but we started treating them like movie skits and we were laughing again.

We knew the battle we were up against, but we adjusted and learned how to handle the issues. We never looked too far ahead and though your progress was very slow and frustrating, there was still progress. We depended on our faith and the belief that we would somehow make it through this time. We had realistic hope for your recovery and we continued thinking, saying, and doing "baby steps, baby steps" over and over again.

12 Stability, Transitions, and Plateaus

March 1993

Dear Jeff,

It was a warmer than usual winter and we welcomed in the New Year with renewed energy and an optimistic attitude. You were feeling pretty good and we were very thankful for a second chance at life. We made plans for a trip, went out to dinner, and did many of the fun things we used to do. You have made a remarkable recovery since June and we both have come a long way. At this time, I would say the word stability best describes the status of my life. I am feeling this way because stability to me means balanced. Nine months ago, I never thought I would ever feel stable or balanced again. The other evening when we were in bed looking through the travel brochures I said, "Jeff, this has been the most stable time I've known since you took ill. I have found an inner peace, there is a balance between us, and I feel harmony in my life." We slowly made our "baby step-by-baby step" transition from one phase of your illness to another. We have reached a plateau where we can rest. We have a good understanding about the disease and there is an accepted and settled feeling with us that is wonderful. The past few months could have destroyed us, but we managed to survive and stabilize. And, we made it together. I never knew what the words cherish every moment meant until now.

From the beginning of our marriage, it could never be described as stable. We were young and naïve when I got pregnant. We were best friends but we were not lovers. You didn't want to marry me because you loved me. You did it because it was the right thing to do. After the miscarriage, we chose to continue trying to make our marriage work. We had interests in common, shared similar goals, values, hopes and dreams. The hurtful part was that I was angry and miserable about my life and you were terribly frustrated by me. You were questioning your sexuality and trying to adjust to a marriage and lifestyle you didn't anticipate. Though I was working and independent, I wanted a certain way of life and the financial security you could provide. These complex, emotional issues caused us to argue a great deal of the time. However, over the years we endured, persevered, and accomplished the goal set out to achieve. We attained the degrees you needed to further your career. We traveled extensively and built several beautiful homes. We always knew what we wanted, but frequently we questioned who we were. On the outside, we appeared confident, secure, and in control of everything we did. "We were the perfect couple who had it all." It was the picture we wanted our family and friends to see. And it was easy for us to be Dr. and Mrs. Jeffrey A. Mintz in the public eye and for your career. You were a handsome successful doctor and I was the beautiful outgoing woman who adored you. Only because of your illness years later, would our family and friends finally learn about the other side of the perfect pair. Behind closed doors, we were living in a fragile, vulnerable co-dependent relationship. "We were stable individuals in an unstable situation." It has taken me a long time to recognize and finally admit that I was unhappy and afraid many times throughout my marriage.

Over the past twenty-three years, we've gone through many transitions that have helped us grow and change, both personally and professionally. We also reached several rewarding and enjoyable plateaus. But, what I've learned recently is that while I was going through these passages, I didn't always recognize they were happening. I overlooked and didn't appreciate the stable times and the comfortable plateaus. I was putting so much stress and pressure on myself because I felt responsible for everything that happened. Maybe these times didn't feel normal because I was too busy searching for something else. Perhaps they were too infrequent to comprehend or not long enough to adjust to. I also know that I was overwhelmed trying to make our difficult marriage work. I am thankful for my renewed sense of appreciation, because I have seen the broader picture with a different perspective. Coming face to face with my past and accepting myself now has been both frightening and empowering. All I focus on now is keeping a balance in the present.

Once you were home and the initial crisis behind us, we needed some stability in our lives more than ever. It would not be easy to achieve because your illness demanded so much energy from us. We knew what we were up against and that your long-term outlook and prognosis wasn't good. If we were both going to recover from this ordeal, we had to have a honeymoon period with the disease. Since our life was changing daily, drastically, and without warning, some of our adjustments were simple and easy, while others were demanding and overwhelming. We never knew when you would react violently to a medication or treatment. Your immune system was severely weakened and many everyday occurrences could become deadly encounters. We learned early on "not to try and take control of the disease that was out of control." Our efforts only proved to be futile and much valuable time and energy would be wasted. You had to become knowledgeable and familiar with the disease and its issues.

We worked harder making endless compromises emotionally, physically, and mentally trying to keep our marriage together. We became more flexible as we adjusted to difficult and challenging situations. We had to learn to manage chaos, understand the difference between sanity and insanity, and recognize that nothing would be normal again. We allowed ourselves to handle the effects of the illness in our own way. We gave ourselves permission to react individually and to make our own choices. We accepted the fact that we coped the best way we could with the skills and techniques we had acquired. We achieved this stability because we focused on what was necessary for your recovery. This balance was frustrating and difficult to accomplish, but we continued going forward facing our challenges.

Because of this terrible tragedy, my perception, interpretation, and appreciation of the word stability had changed. Stability now signified a day that was quiet without a medical crisis. It could be a week when you were feeling stronger, tolerating your treatments and medications. Stable could be a month when you were exercising again, regaining your energy and having quality of life. Stable was a nine-month respite from the pneumonia. Though our progress was slow and rocky, we eventually reached our goal and a plateau. The long transition period during your recovery was worthwhile because it helped strengthen our relationship. We were overwhelmed and overjoyed with feelings of fulfillment and accomplishment. I've become more aware of the importance of the words stability, plateaus, and transitions. I also understand that the most stressful and disruptive times can prove to be the most productive and powerful ones.

In May 1993, you became ill with your second PCP infection. While in the hospital with you, I heard an expression that seemed appropriate for this time.

"Stability is but a fleeting moment when in fact there is nothing stable at all." We had reached a plateau with the disease during the past year that we had gotten comfortable with. We had adjusted to our situation, but within twenty-four hours our world was turned upside down in turmoil again. We were now dealing with an entirely different set of circumstances. We had to regroup and refocus, continuously making new decisions about your condition. We were frightened, not knowing the outcome. Because it took longer for you to recover and your progress was much slower, our adjustments took longer to make and our frustrations were more excruciating and overwhelming than ever. With this second pneumonia, the duration of time with stability, plateaus, and transitions continued to get shorter, became less frequent, more difficult to understand, and much harder to deal with.

In 1994, you developed your third and final bout with pneumonia. I remember the morning in May when you gave me a look. Your eyes said something I had never seen before. You were losing the long difficult battle and you didn't want to fight any longer. You felt you had nothing left to fight for. Your days were painful. You didn't have any quality of life.

Your illness had taken its toll on everyone you loved and everyone that loved you. You wanted to end your suffering and made one last decision. You were going to leave your last plateau and make your final transition with Hospice help. As your body was letting go and shutting down, Hospice was here with us giving our life stability and balance. They helped you make this transition easier, more humane, and dignified.

What is the most difficult thing for me to admit now is that I know there were times when I could have enjoyed myself more and been happier. I was in the middle of my own personal nightmare and I would not allow myself to wake up. I tried to take charge of everything in my life for so long. I wanted life to be the way I thought it should be. So, my darling, our life was a series of transitions and plateaus. But, recognizing, understanding, and accepting them are what's important. I used to think that the only way to reach a plateau was to go uphill. It wasn't until you became ill that I realized some plateaus go downhill also. However, the speed going downhill is much quicker than the pace climbing up. Reaching an uphill plateau took you so long, but you went downhill very quickly. Your first transition felt like it took forever, but your final one was very short. But, once I understood what this precious thing called life was really all about, I found stability in the instability. I discovered plateaus everywhere I went, and transitions that didn't have to go anywhere. I made a transition into a new way of thinking bringing a balance and peaceful feeling I hope will continue.

August 1, 1994

Dear Jeff,

"Honey, I'm so afraid. Who's going to take care of me?" Since the beginning of our marriage, I have been dependent upon you for so many things. How many times has this issue forced me to come face to face with my worst fears? Though I have always dreaded your possible answer, for the past twenty-three years, I've never been able to avoid asking you this question. Before you took ill, whenever I brought this subject up, my heart beat furiously in anxious anticipation of your response. But, it wasn't until your diagnosis on June 19th, that I realized how significant the impact and depth of my insecurity would truly be. I know that you only have a few weeks longer to live and I don't know what to do. My heart aches for you and the pain of this horrible ordeal tears at my soul. I am in the depths of despair, terrified, and panicked about my future without you. Tonight, for the very last time, I will ask you the question, "Who will take care of me?"

I was sitting on the side of the bed resting my head on your frail and tired body. I took your beautiful hands in mine and said, "Jeff, who will take care of me?" This time you knew from the tone of my voice that I desperately needed your support and reassurance. You could barely speak and your brown eyes were intensely focused on mine. You took a deep breath and very slowly said, "Bee, you'll be fine. You'll take care of yourself. You'll have friends and you'll live your life the way you always have. You are a strong, confident, beautiful woman who can do anything you set your mind to. I'll always take care of you and I'll always be with you. It just won't be the way it is now." I collapsed emotionally, crying hysterically, out of control on your chest. I wanted to die along with you. I could not bear to think of my life without you. You held me so close, continuing to reassure me that I would be all right. Your belief and faith in me was overwhelming and overpowering. I fell asleep on your body and awoke to the phone announcing that our Hospice aide was here for the night. I went into the other room and tried to sleep, but my mind continued to race with unanswerable questions about an uncertain and frightening future. Your words played over and over again in my mind, but your assurances could not lessen my fears.

From the time we met in the fifth grade, we immediately became best friends. It was easy because our friendship was based on fun, laughter, and great communication. We instinctively knew each other and it was apparent early on that something very special and meaningful was happening between us. You were thoughtful and considerate, constantly thinking about what I liked or what made me happy. When I was sick, you babied me and played "nurse." When I was sad, you could cheer me up with your silly antics and wonderful sense of humor. You could make me laugh like nobody else could. When I had doubts or was fearful and frustrated, you were patient and sensitive to my concerns. You gave me your unconditional support and friendship. You enjoyed making my birthdays and our anniversaries memorable events with unexpected surprises and beautiful gifts. You were class with a five-star rating when it came to appreciating the finer things in life. You planned our wonderful trips, bought all the tickets to the theater, ballet, and opera. And how we loved going to movies. How many times did we go to see three in one day? We called them our cinema fix. You also derived great pleasure from shopping and sought out every opportunity to indulge in your purchasing passion. You mother continuously told you that the only reason we had any money was because I was so frugal. I liked keeping a watchful eye on our finances and you respected me for that. We had fun making plans, setting goals, and completing whatever we set out to accomplish.

However, my concerns about who will take care of me had been a constant issue that had troubled me throughout my life. I was an insecure, frustrated, and unhappy twenty-two year old when we married. Maybe I was weak, immature, and vulnerable, but you were the kind of man I'd always dreamed of marrying. You had impeccable taste. You were charming, handsome, and intelligent. You would have been successful in anything you ever wanted to do. You were a wonderful devoted son, a trusted friend, and a caring sensitive person. You made me feel safe, secure, and confident about myself. You were proud of the things I did and you loved my intensity, passion, and the power of my convictions. You cared about the person I was and who I wanted to be. You were my rock emotionally, spiritually, and mentally. You gave me honest opinions, sound advice, and guidance. You had a way of putting everything in order. These marvelous qualities were just a few of the many reasons I loved you and continued to stay married to you. Money was also an important issue to me and I knew you would provide the financial security I wanted. If you were able to give me the things that mattered the most to me, why shouldn't I benefit from this opportunity?

So, was I a naïve young girl who thought she was in love or was I really an insecure and dependent woman? Did I stay with you for the right reasons or was I lying and deceiving myself? Did I give in to your interests and bisexual lifestyle because I was afraid to get divorced and go out into the world alone? Was it easier to compromise myself for the good life that you could provide? Was I the perfect partner for someone like you because I didn't want to be on my own and was afraid about many things in my life? Through my writing and after much self-analysis, I was finally able to understand the issues that fueled these troublesome questions. You wanted to take care of me and that's what I wanted you to do. We accepted our co-dependency upon each other, made our own decisions, and we chose to take care of each other. Our relationship worked because we both knew what we were doing. We understood our motives and the reasons why we were staying together. We balanced each other perfectly and together we were a powerful team. However, over the years I was developing an unhealthy negative pattern of behavior and my dependency upon you was becoming like an addiction. My insecurity became a trend that continued to be one of the most dominant factors influencing our marriage. I know now that I would never have had the strength and courage to walk away from you or our marriage. I needed to stay married to you no matter what the price.

We became dependent upon one another as we continued to build our life together. But whenever I was faced with a situation or had to make a decision involving the security of my financial future, I asked myself the who will take care of me question. When you wanted to go to school in Gainesville, I immediately said, "When do we move?" And why wouldn't I feel this way? In three years you would graduate and become a doctor. You would be able to financially take care of me. I wouldn't have to work any longer, and I would be able to pursue other interests. After our move to Houston, we established your private practice and you were finally in a position to give me all the things I'd ever dreamed of. I had the freedom and the time to enjoy my new life and the money to do whatever I wanted. Our final move to Boca Raton was the culmination of sixteen years of hard work and teamwork. I admit honestly and openly that you spoiled me, took exceptional care of me, and would have done anything you could to make me happy. You would never stop taking care of me because you always had.

Tonight, I am not the insecure girl you married who was caught up in the illusion of a comfortable lifestyle. I have become a mature woman whose fears concerning her own inadequacies have lessened. My focus now and my fears have shifted to you as my husband, your bisexual lifestyle, and your possible battle with a deadly disease. After I heard about AIDS, the who will take care of me question took on a different, more terrifying new meaning. When you eventually became ill, again my question did not change, but the horrifying answer did. Now, your impending death has me paralyzed in terror. I fear as a loving devoted wife who is going to lose her husband. As your long-time companion and loyal friend, I am afraid as I watch my life partner of twenty-five years die. The who will take care of me question is the same, but the answers and the reasons for them have changed. I am going to have to take care of myself, because you will no longer be here to take care of me. I will be on my own for the first time in twenty-five years thrown into a lifestyle that will be unfamiliar and disturbing.

I am not ashamed to say that I needed you because you were always there to take care of me. When it came to being responsible, dependable, and reliable, you never once failed me. I needed your honesty, support, understanding, and your unconditional acceptance of our love. And I wanted the financial and emotional security that you could provide as my husband and friend. I have learned many valuable lessons during our marriage and most recently because of your illness. During our past two years together, I've come to realize I was stronger than I thought I was. I have become a more confident and secure woman because I am able to face this crisis with you. Your trust and faith in me at this time has helped me gain a self-directed confidence I didn't know I had. I now believe the who will take care of me person has finally become the I will take care of me woman. Through your tears and weakening voice, on August 1st, 1994, you were right when you said to me, "Bee, you will take care of yourself." In fact, I know now that I had been doing exactly that throughout my entire marriage. However, it was something that took a long time for me to figure out and I had to learn about it through my own experiences. Of one thing I am deadly certain, I know I took care of you, you took care of me and we took care of each other.

14 Facing my Fears and Future as a Widow

"I will take the time to let the time take care of me. Perhaps it was fate, destiny, or chance, but we would never give up on each other or our relationship."

Dear Jeff,

At this moment I am barely coping with your impending fate. I doubt my life and my reasons for living. I am unsure of what I will be able to deal with or how I am going to survive the months following your death. This uncertainty now has me torn apart and I cannot comprehend where I will get the strength to go on. Though I know you are dying and I am going to be alone, my future without you has not yet happened. You are still alive and we will continue to share our life together until death do us part. We must wait and hope that your final days are as peaceful and comfortable as possible. A part of me is in denial and does not want to accept a future without you, while another part is brutally aware and accepting of it. I am caught up in the middle of this horrible conflict. I am searching deeply within myself trying to understand the most frightening things that I cannot possibly imagine. What I will do without you?

My greatest pleasure and rewards came from taking care of our home. I loved being your partner. My world revolved around you, your career and the life we made together. My days with you were filled with passion, excitement, and fun. I was addicted to the adventure you added to my life. You gave me direction and helped me to focus on what was important. How will I ever be able to walk into our home again, or eat at the kitchen table, or sleep in our bed without you? Who will I cook for? Will I ever be able to go to the movies alone or watch our annual beauty pageants without crying? How will I ever be able to go to the beach, walk in the sand, watch beautiful sunsets, or enjoy the flight of a pelican overhead? What will I do on my birthday and anniversary? Who will tell me they are proud of me and that I am special? Who will buy me fragrant perfumes, flowers, or pretty clothes? Who will I travel with and share those fun-filled exotic trips? What will I do for the holidays and other festive occasions when family and friends are all around? Who will be honest and encourage me to pursue my dreams and help me accomplish my goals? Who will hold me when I am cold at night or make me a cup of tea or cook dinner for me when I get ill? Will I ever be happy and smile again? Will I ever be able to rid my mind of the horrible images I see before me? Will I withdraw into a solitary world of memories? Will I give up the things I used to do as I try to accept new and unfamiliar challenges? How much of my life will I have to change and will I be able to accept these changes? Oh, Jeff, what will I do without you?

I am too young and alive to become a widow. It does not feel right or make any sense. I wanted to spend the rest of my life with you. We were supposed to grow old together and no one or nothing was going to change the picture I had in my mind. That was the way it was supposed to be. We were a team. We still had so many more wonderful things to accomplish and experience. Our parents were still alive. We had many interesting and fun-loving friends, and we had a lifetime of exciting adventures to look forward to. You have given me everything I have always dreamed of. How could I ask for anything more? You are the one I was supposed to share all of this with.

What good is the time and money if we can't enjoy it together? Though our life together was unconventional, we made the marriage work because we never gave up on each other. We had our share of problems, but every relationship does. Somehow, we always managed to talk it out. It's ironic that I hadn't told you this until now, but did you know that before you took ill our relationship was the best it had ever been? I had accepted our tumultuous and passionate relationship because I wanted to stay married to you. I learned to live with your bisexuality and understood that it had nothing to do with us. You were the way you were and I would not try to change you. We had our life together, but we also had our own individual lives. I was involved with my writing career. I had developed my own interests, friends, and goals I wanted to fulfill. I had become someone I liked and respected because I was handling my life with you in an honest and healthy manner. But, you were the core that gave everything in my life meaning and purpose. My life meant something because our life together meant everything. Why should this disease take you from me at a time in my life when I wanted and needed you the most? What will I do without you?

On July 4th, 1994, just two years after I brought you home from the hospital, I will ask you a terrifying question that I have never dared ask of you before. I didn't have to deal with it until now and I also couldn't find the courage and strength to face it. However, if I am going to get through this horrible time, I must address this painful issue with you now. I have no choice. I do not ask you this question because I am insecure, immature, and dependent upon you. I am asking you this as your wife, best friend, and devoted longtime companion. My question is based on wants not needs. As I sit next to your bed tonight stroking your forehead, I cannot avoid asking you this any longer. "Jeff, what will I do without you?" For a few moments we sat in silence, both of us painfully aware of the impact this question had. You took my trembling hands in yours and with a gentle loving voice said, "Susan, take it one day at a time remembering who you are and what you have become. You will eventually go back to your routine and do the same things you loved to do. Only now, you will do them without me. You will allow different people into your life and you'll explore your feelings deeply and honestly. You will handle your life the way you always have and continue to grow in strength and with courage. You will take on exciting challenges and share wonderful experiences with others. You will go on and become stronger and happier than you have ever been. You will do this because this is the way you are. You will miss me, but eventually you will welcome and embrace your new life. You will have an identity and a life all your own. You will be everything you ever wanted to be and I will be with you. I will always be there with you. I promise you this."

On January 11th, 1969, I made my unconditional commitment to you. I made the decision to love you with all my heart and soul for the rest of my life. It wasn't a duty or an obligation. It was a choice. I would have compromised anything to keep you in my life, and I would have done whatever I had to do in order to make our marriage work. My marriage was difficult, but it was mine. My life with you was turbulent, but it was my life. I knew if the marriage was not successful, our enduring friendship would have been strong enough to keep us together. We both knew we were worth the extra effort and we would never have given up on us. I can honestly tell you now I know you would never have left me. I remember joking with you, dozens of times, stating why I knew you would never leave me. You loved my cooking and the way I did your laundry, especially your shirts. I kidded with you about this and many other things until now. And you had to feel the same way because you were the one having the sexual encounters with men. You had many opportunities to leave me, but you always chose to come back. Though it was horribly difficult, I learned how to accept your homosexual desires as a part of our lifestyle, and I understood your passions and your needs. You know I never felt threatened or felt like I had to compete with these men. They were temporary partners who came and went in and out of your life. You were two ships passing in the night. But, what will I do without your friendship? Because that is the one thing we always shared that I could count on. I will miss the friendship the most.

On June 19, 1992, a part of me buried you along with your diagnosis. Though I feel like I am dying along with you, I know I am not. Tonight my darling, as the fireworks light up the moonlit sky, I asked for your guidance, your support, and your reassurance. And as it had been throughout our marriage, you were right. You told me what I needed to hear and I am hopeful and comforted by the faith you have in me. You made me believe that one day I would be all right. I was afraid to ask you my question because of what I would hear, but as I lie awake in my bed tonight, I know that I will slowly adjust. I will settle into a new life with different people, places, and things. I will go on as others have done before me. I will learn to do my future without the man I was accustomed to sharing my life with. But, I know I will be all right if I take the time to let the time take care of me. You were my partner, my friend, and my forever love. What will I do without you? I will do all right because you will always be with me.

15 Long Term Plans, Short Term Goals

"Many times, I didn't know if the truth was a lie or the lie was the truth." Susan Lee Mintz

Dear Jeff,

We faced the demanding challenges of your illness for two years. We succeeded because we never stopped compromising as problems and obstacles came our way. We learned that making plans would still be easy, but having them turn out the way we expected or anticipated would be another matter. Something once simple and fun now became extremely difficult or nearly impossible. We had to radically change our perception of what long-term versus short-term meant. The words daily living now took on a cruel and brutal new meaning. Planning something three months in advance might have to be canceled within twenty-four hours, because without warning we could be faced with a crisis or medical emergency. We had to evaluate and question everything we wanted to do, and we never had the luxury of planning long-term again. We learned how to live day to day and moment to moment as everything around us changed drastically and quickly.

I called you Daniel Boone because even as a teenager traveling was your passion. You loved planning trips and were always visiting fun and interesting places. Whether skiing a challenging mountain or sunning on a distant beach, you were different and exciting. After we married, you made it perfectly clear I was going to be your navigator. You took AAA books and maps to bed, falling asleep with pen and magic marker in hand. You went into a hypnotic state while making our hotel and restaurant reservations. You planned car trips to California, Seattle, and Canada solely around restaurants, art galleries, and museums and you bought tickets for everything. We went to Spain on our honeymoon. We visited Caracas, Europe, Mexico, and all the Caribbean Islands. I spent four wonderful birthdays in a row in Hawaii. You enjoyed every aspect of traveling and you loved sharing your exciting adventurous life with me. My biggest decisions were what to wear and how many suitcases to take. You planned our trips six months in advance, and in twenty-three years we never canceled or postponed one of them. You were known at the airports, on the planes, and in the hotels and restaurants. Because of your work with the military and oil companies, we took many luxurious vacations as a fringe benefit.

After the pneumonia in June 1992, it took you six months to recover and regain your strength. Even as you got stronger and were able to travel again, you still tired easily. It was obvious that you would not be able to travel the way you did before. This issue was one of the most devastating and depressing ones you had to face. We now took everything we did one day at a time. We had to be prepared, organized, and never took any chances. We could have problems with the weather, eating and sleeping accommodations, car reservations, or airline postponements. Whether it was going to a movie that same day or planning a trip three months later, our plans could change quickly without warning. You got tired, nauseous, and had diarrhea for days. You spiked 104-degree fevers and became delirious. Sometimes you couldn't eat, drink, or even breathe. You were taking several medications that had serious side effects. Your immune system was compromised and you were prone to numerous infections that could require immediate medical attention.

I was the one who had to find the doctors, hospitals, or make the arrangements to get you home if you took ill. Before any trip, I packed a bag full of pills, creams, sprays, preventive secondary prescriptions, and referral names for other doctors. I carried extra supplies with us and wrote down everything in a journal. We kept an address book with our doctor's names and phone numbers. We started taking cruises to Bermuda and the Caribbean Islands because they were safer and more controlled. The first time we took out cancellation insurance, it was a bitter reminder of your precarious condition. Cruising was not the way you wanted to travel and I know you did this to make it easier for me. You never stopped wanting the spontaneous excitement of the life you once loved. But, that effortless travel we used to enjoy had become a difficult task both mentally and physically.

By January 1993, you were strong enough to travel again. We decided to go to New York for a week to visit my parents. Our flight was scheduled for March 15th. We would rent a car, stay in a motel apartment, and visit with family and friends. My parents loved you like a son and wanted to see you so badly. Two days before the trip, you ran a low-grade fever and developed a dry hacking cough. These symptoms could indicate the beginning of a simple cold or the start of pneumonia. My parents called stating it was bitterly cold and that a blizzard was expected. You insisted on going and I got hysterical. I was terrified and screamed, "How can we go if you're getting ill?" You finally canceled the trip, but it was the first time we ever fought over travel plans. We took our frustrations out on each other and it was horrible. Three days later, you developed a bronchial infection, but it wasn't pneumonia. We rescheduled for March 26th and this time we made it. You looked wonderful. Your attitude was incredibly positive, and no one other than my parents knew you were ill.

The trip exhausted you and we canceled a cruise for April. However, you started planning a trip to our favorite country, Italy. You wanted to be in Amalfi on May 4th for my 48th birthday. Sadly, we both knew this might be the last trip we would take. You made the arrangements mapping out a fourteen-day motor trip starting in Rome and ending in Venice. We would visit ancient exciting cities, eat delicious foods, and spend romantic nights in charming picturesque hotels. Two days before the trip, I got frightened. Would this be too much for you? What would I do if you took ill in a country halfway around the world? I worried about fatigue and the demands of driving and sightseeing. We didn't speak the language. We would have a car with a standard shift that I didn't know how to drive. Would you be able to take care of me if I took ill?

However, we arrived in Rome and you felt better than you had in a while. The hotel was magnificent, and on May 4th, 1994, we were in Amalfi, Italy, under a breathtaking full moon. We strolled arm in arm down the small winding street to the quaint little family restaurant. You gave me a card, perfume, and said you loved me more than ever before. All my fears and horrible thoughts that haunted me before the trip were gone. We gazed into each other's eyes as we shared a delicious home cooked meal. It was the ultimate adventure and something we had to prove to ourselves. I was in awe of your strength, attitude, and your love for life. It was the most beautiful birthday I ever had.

A week later while heading towards our hotel in Tuscany, we had a terrible scare. Our car overheated and for two hours we were stranded in the middle of nowhere. It was cold and we didn't have any food or water. You were tired, coughing, and needed to take your medication. Finally, a truck driver stopped and though he didn't speak English and we didn't speak Italian, one hour later our radiator was filled with coolant. We made it to the hotel fifty miles away. When we arrived, they didn't have our reservation. I pleaded with the English-speaking manager telling him you were seriously ill. Eventually, he found us a small room but stated the heater was broken. At this point, we didn't care. You were exhausted and needed to eat and rest. Rome was several hours away and if you took ill now, I didn't know what I would do. The room was freezing. We held each other under several quilts, but never did sleep. However, in the morning you felt better and we continued on our journey. You bought me beautiful clothes in Milan and magnificent glass in Venice. We visited the Isle of Capri, Florence, Pisa, and Sienna. We laughed and cried a lot during those two weeks as we shared twenty-five years of memories. After returning home, we agreed it was the best trip we had ever taken.

It took weeks for you to regain your strength. Your resistance was low and you had constant low-grade fevers. But you wanted to take another trip. You were the senior class president at American International College in Springfield, Massachusetts, and it was your twenty-fifth year reunion. As president, you wanted to attend. We decided we would fly to Albany, visit my parents, and drive to Springfield. You reserved a suite at the hotel and sent out twenty-five invitations to fraternity brothers inviting them to a private party on Friday night. You had lost weight, but when you got dressed up, you looked wonderful. We spent a few days with my parents and drove to Springfield on Friday. We stopped to get supplies for the party. By the time we got to the hotel, you had a violent attack of diarrhea and a 102-degree fever. I thought you were getting a bacterial infection and begged you to cancel the party.

You said you would not change your plans. You took two Tylenol and bundled up under several blankets. An hour later, you broke a sweat that drenched the sheets. You asked me to get dressed and be the perfect wife and hostess because your brothers would soon arrive. You were feeling better, took a shower, and when you came out, they never suspected a thing. You were as handsome and charming as your friends remembered twenty-five years ago. I played my part well and had become very good at hiding the truth, along with my feelings. It was a wonderful night and at 1:00 AM, we collapsed in bed. You spiked another fever, took two Tylenol and broke a sweat at 4:00 AM. You woke up early and went to the college to visit teachers and colleagues. The formal black tie dinner was tonight and you were the keynote speaker. It would be difficult to me to pretend that nothing was wrong because you were definitely not feeling well. I didn't know if you would make it through the night. But, as you gave your speech in front of 150 classmates, you were incredible. How could someone so deathly ill be so inspiring and have that much control? As we said our good-byes, we knew we accomplished something that had to be done. You went back to the hotel seriously ill and we flew home from Springfield the next day.

We went immediately to the hospital and you were diagnosed with a third bout of pneumonia. "We gave up everything, but we gave up nothing." From June 19, 1992, until August 17, 1994, we enjoyed many wonderful trips. We learned to adjust to the challenges as we lived with AIDS. We worked around the disease and we rearranged our life as it progressed. We cherished every moment knowing that the only thing we could control was the way we handled this time. We learned to be flexible and didn't hide our fears. This illness tested us at every level and could have either destroyed us or made our relationship stronger. I know one thing for sure, we were a great team. In the end, we proved to ourselves that we had beaten the odds and we won.

16 . Jeff Comforted Me, I Comforted Him, We Comforted Each Other

"Many times it was impossible to determine which one of us was the caregiver or which one was the patient."

Dear Jeff,

We hated studying and were terrible students in high school. It was our junior year and we were the only Jewish kids to fail three subjects. We had to attend summer school and if we didn't pass all the subjects, we would not have graduated the following year. It was the summer of 1963, we were seventeen years old and spent all our time together, studying, talking, and laughing. It was one of the best summers of my life. Summer school brought us together and solidified the friendship that continued over the years. In 1990, when I wrote my cookbook, you laughed at me because you couldn't understand how someone who didn't like to read could be such a good writer. I said, "it was a gift that somehow just happened." I still do not read, but on June 19, 1992, when I started journaling, I learned to become very comfortable with a dictionary and thesaurus. My writing has enabled me to come to terms with difficult issues and handle my personal problems. It has also given me the comfort and support I needed when no one or nothing else could.

Since you have taken ill, there are two words that I find myself thinking about quite frequently. These words are comfort and support. When I looked their meaning up, I found out that these words can mean the same thing and are interchangeable. Comfort as a verb means to give hope, to console, or show sympathy and compassion in times of fear or grief. Comfort as a noun means a state of ease or well-being, encouragement, help, or support. Over the years, we shared these meanings many times both together and independently. At times, we were uncertain which one of us was the patient or the caregiver. Until the situation presented itself, we never knew which one would be the stronger of the two. As partners in a marriage, there were times when we needed to comfort each other. If our marriage was a give and take, there were times when one of us gave more comfort than the other one did. If the words commitment and marriage mean sharing both the best and worst of times, then we definitely unconditionally comforted and supported each other through this difficult period. And, whether we were giving or receiving comfort, both of us did a lot of both.

During your illness nothing was going to be easy, predictable, or consistent. As we continued learning how to cope with this time, I compared it to an endless dance of heightened emotions and super charged feelings. That explanation gave me something I could picture and base my feelings upon. The choreographer of this dance was love. We were the partners dancing though this time with the feelings of comfort and support guiding us both separately and together. One of us led, keeping the beat to an emotional rhythm while the other partner followed. At other times, our roles changed and the leader became the follower. We continued to alternate our emotional strengths and weaknesses. Many times as we danced as a team, we knew the steps and followed each other's leads. We were totally aware of each other's feelings knowing when to hold each other, console one another, or perhaps leave each other alone. However, there were times when both of us remained motionless though the music continued. We practiced a lot during this time and the more involved we got with the illness, the better we were. Whether we danced emotionally together, apart, or sometimes not at all, it was our dance of life for two years with AIDS. As we questioned our ability to continue performing during this marathon time, it was our comfort and support that gave us the strength to go on.

From 1981 through 1992, we learned that rationalizing was a very effective way for us to comfort each other. Rationalizing worked because we were able to find a comfortable place to store our hard to face unresolved issues. If we didn't have to face a problem, then we wouldn't have to solve it. With many of our friends in Houston dying from AIDS, we knew this disease threatened our lives. Yet, we continually rationalized your lifestyle, your bisexuality, and your lovers. I told you that you couldn't get AIDS, because you were "married to the perfect homemaker." You said you were too healthy, happy, and had everything in life to live for. You laughed saying it wasn't in our future, because we were going to grow old together. We talked about the subject, supported and comforted each other, and always managed put it out of our minds. But, we were deceiving ourselves because this disease was never out of our minds. All we did was give ourselves a false sense of security. We learned how to tuck the issue neatly away in a private place that enabled us to live with it. Why should we worry about something that might never happen?

But, I never comforted you more than on June 19, 1992, when you were diagnosed. As you faced your mortality with this deadly disease, you needed to know your quality of life and dignity were always my priority. You continually said, "Susan, no matter what happens, please make sure I die the way I lived." You needed my physical comfort when your fevers spiked to 104 degrees. I wrapped extra blankets around your shaking body and laid on top of you until the fever broke. You needed my emotional support as I held you in my arms reassuring you that one day you would feel better. I comforted you when I told you I loved you and that we would fight this disease together. And you needed my support the most when I said I would never let anything happen to you. You needed my words of encouragement, the strength of my body and mind, and my unconditional commitment to you. I know, my darling, that you would have done the same for me.

As a comforting wife and supportive friend, the most horrible times for me happened when I fell apart in front of you. However, these were the times that enabled me to open up the most and be honest about my feelings. Eventually, my break down weaknesses gave me strength. Once I allowed myself to face my humanness and fragility, I became more effective and supportive for you. I started to understand the fact that my strength, determination, and confidence would continually be tested. I realized I might not be able to live up to my own expectations and I handled my life as two separate women. I had two different personalities and conducted myself according to the role I had to play. As Susan your friend, I was confident, controlled, and always in command of the situation. I was emotionally disciplined and precise about what had to be done. When I was Susan your wife, I was vulnerable, easily affected, and never as strong as I wanted to be. But, as your spouse, I could break down and tell you that I was also afraid. I fell apart so many times as I watched you suffer with this disease. I'd make up an excuse to leave the room, because it was too painful for me to watch you try to eat. When I heard you tossing in bed all night my heart ached. I would be driving along when I'd hear a song that reminded me of something we shared. I would have to pull off to the side of the road because I would get hysterical and wouldn't be able to see through my tears. As couples walked hand in hand on the beach, I knew we would never share this special time again. At times like this, my writing was my comfort and support.

We needed to support and comfort each other when you got your lab results back. Your blood work and counts were always out of the normal range and when you saw these results you panicked. This frightened me also and together, we were reminded of how seriously ill you were. Our hearts raced before your doctors' appointments and chest x-rays. We supported each other as we dealt with the frustrations of your medications. You had to take some with food, others at bedtime, and many were so large they had to be crushed. We cried together because of your diminished appetite. I made you delicious meals and you tried forcing yourself to eat, but couldn't. You coughed, got nauseous, or had no energy. And we desperately needed to support each other as we watched this disease waste your beautiful body away.

This was the cruelest thing for you because there was nothing we could do about it. I constantly told you, "Jeff, you are still the handsomest man I've ever known. Your smile melts my heart just as it did the first time I saw you." We comforted each other as you became more dependent and everything you were was gradually slipping away. Finally, when it came to the issue of your parents, we needed to comfort and support them because we knew the pain they would be dealing with. I had to reassure you they would be taken care of.

And then there were the times when you were the stronger one giving me comfort and support. I lost control so easily and for many reasons. I'd break down over a phone call, a lab report, or a doctor's opinion. You knew my concerns about your parents, the medical bills, and my own health. Where did you find this strength to comfort me? Many times you were my caregiver and your strength, reassuring words, and encouragement temporarily managed to convince me that everything would be all right. You tried to lessen my sadness because you knew your illness was my illness too. Your strength was my inspiration. You constantly told me I was "your Godsend" and you couldn't do this without me. You comforted me as a friend, a woman, and as your wife who was suffering along with her husband. You supported me when I was afraid for myself and the uncertainty of a future alone. You comforted me when I couldn't watch your pain any longer and screamed out loud because this wasn't fair. You understood how difficult this time was for me. Your words of consolation gave me permission and allowed me to let go.

From January 11, 1969, until August 17,1994, we gave each other unconditional comfort and support physically, mentally, emotionally, and spiritually. And for twenty-five years, we were giving care and taking care of each other. We were both weak and strong as we faced our life and this tragic time together. We were a team who balanced each other whether giving or receiving comfort and support. We had shared a life that was tumultuous and chaotic, but it was a wonderful life full of choices, ups and downs, passion, and love. You gave me my reason to live and I never had any regrets. I am glad you allowed me to give you care. Take care, my love.

17 Frustrations, Setbacks, and Disappointments

"Will I be strong enough for you and find the courage within myself for me?"

"The only choices we had were how we were going to handle our choices."

Dear Jeff,

If the expression, "with age comes wisdom" is true, hopefully one day I might consider myself a wise person. But, how much wisdom does someone need to be considered wise? If life is an accumulation of learning experiences, will I become more insightful, courageous, and gain a deeper inner strength as my evolutionary process continues? There were many times during our marriage when I questioned and doubted some of my decisions. It has taken your illness for me to recognize and absolutely unconditionally believe that from the time we got married every choice I made was the right one. Does my acknowledgment of the feelings of fulfillment and gratification give me permission to consider myself a wise woman? Or is my age of wisdom just beginning? Is my awakening going to grant me more patience with others and with myself in the future? Has my maturity allowed me to both recognize and admit that disappointments, frustrations, and setbacks are an important yet terribly difficult part of life's learning process? My most heart breaking disappointment is that very soon we will not be facing any more hurdles and obstacles together.

I think happiness or unhappiness has nothing to do with being optimistic. I've maintained a positive attitude about life, though many times I've been unhappy. Over the years, through the best and worst of situations, there is one word that has empowered and challenged me. Though it has been a strong and courageous ally through my darkest hours, it has also been a fierce and cruel adversary. The word is NO and its meaning can be one of life's most difficult reality checks. If my life under normal circumstances has been frustrating and challenging, how will I manage to maintain a positive attitude through this dreadful time? Will I be sensitive, intuitive, and wise enough to accept the setbacks of your illness? Will I accept my fate because it is part of a bigger picture? Will I be able to handle our ordeal because I am supposed to? Will I continue to be optimistic when I feel there are times I have failed myself and now possibly you? Do I question myself with such intense scrutiny that the decision I make must be the right one? As we face this disease together, will I be strong enough for you and positive enough for us?

Did you know the most difficult times in my life were also my most productive? I believed setbacks were growing experiences I could work through and learn from. I perceived my problems as opportunities that gave me courage and made me stronger. But, what setback could be more horrifying than your diagnosis? What possible challenges could test me more than those devastating words on June 19th? How difficult would our future decisions be as we faced monumental negativity and rejection? How supportive would I be as I watched you suffer from an illness that has destroyed our life? When you become unable to care for yourself, would I be strong enough to take care of you? Would I have the courage to believe in myself? Would I remain hopeful and positive as the disease progresses? We had to depend on and trust other people's opinions, new medications, and frightening issues about life and death. Our setbacks went hand in hand with doctor appointments, x-rays, lab tests, and drug treatments. It was easier for me to focus on something positive during the first few weeks of your illness. I had hopeful expectations and realistic goals. Maybe I was in shock or perhaps just relieved, but my determination to get you well kept me going. Focusing on this issue gave me strength and helped me stay positive. But, how would I remain optimistic and deal with my frustrations now that I shared my life with AIDS?

We did have some things to be positive about. We had excellent health insurance with the best care available. We trusted your doctors who were experts in the fields. Their honest opinions never deceived us with false hope. Though we were knowledgeable about AIDS, we quickly learned we knew very little. We familiarized ourselves with the newest drugs, treatments, and data. Sometimes this information gave us hope because the drugs you received extended your quality of life. However, there were times when our hope vanished because their side effects caused you further suffering. Your frustration caused you to question whether the treatment was worse than the disease. A major setback occurred when you became allergic to Bactrim, a sulfur drug inhibiting the PCP bacteria. How many people did we know who took this common inexpensive pill? When given this drug as a prophylactic treatment, you became deathly ill and were rushed back to the hospital. Since you couldn't tolerate this medication, the only options available involved weekly inhalation treatments and powerful toxic drugs. You were dependent on the medications and owned by the disease.

We desperately wanted to believe a miracle might happen, but in our hearts we knew there were none. Ironically, many times it was our positive attitude that set us up for this frustration. You felt good for several days and your confidence and attitude improved. Then, without warning you wouldn't feel well and all the progress you had made was gone. These setbacks, along with the difficult questions involving your medications, were devastating for you. One day the doctor said you were doing great, but two hours later, a lab report indicated a low white blood cell count or anemia. One minute, we had hope and a moment later, we were disappointed. I remember waiting for a new drug called Mepron to get approved by the FDA. Our doctor said within twenty-four hours of its release, we would have this "miracle drug." It cost $3.00 a pill and you had to take nine of them a day with fatty foods. The possibility of liver failure went along with the price. But, we were willing to try anything to keep you alive. It was approved and the prescription was called into our usual pharmacy. They told me it would be forty-eight hours before they could have it available. With a life-threatening illness, forty-eight hours is a lifetime. This disappointment was horrible to endure. This drug was our only hope and sometimes hope was all we had. I called every drug store from Boca Raton to Miami, finally locating one in Ft. Lauderdale that had received it. I drove like a maniac for two hours in traffic so that you could start on it immediately.

With every attempt we had hope and with every hope came disappointment. The frustration became unbearable as we continued giving up things we once enjoyed. I cannot explain the sadness you endured when you retired from a career you loved and a business you started. When you couldn't exercise, travel, enjoy food, and do the things you loved to do, it was heartbreaking. If there was a chance that something would work and get you better, you tried it. You did alternative treatments including Chinese herbs, acupuncture, aromatherapy, relaxation techniques, juicing, megavitamin treatments, and massages. With every treatment, book, tape, or video, we prayed for anything that would keep you alive until a cure was found. As we rescheduled appointments, waited for unfilled prescriptions, redid lost blood tests, or retook x-rays, our setbacks were endless. The only way we kept ourselves positive was by speaking openly and honestly about everything. We cried with each other and for each other, and we shared this time with our family, friends, and faith.

Whenever we watched a movie, television program, or read an article about something pertaining to AIDS, our hearts skipped a beat. Would we hear something encouraging about a cure or vaccine? No! The news was never good and our disappointments continued. When you heard Arthur Ashe had died, you completely lost control. I was terrified and called the doctor. You couldn't catch your breath and nearly passed out. When we went to see the movie Philadelphia, we both got hysterical. Any issue involving a sensitive subject could upset us. Sometimes we wanted to talk about everything else besides AIDS. We wanted our friends and family to treat us like they did before. But, that didn't happen. We weren't like we were before. People meant well, but their first question was, "Jeff, how are you doing? How are you feeling? You look wonderful." You would say, "I wish my insides looked as good as my outsides." We were constantly being reminded about your illness. How many times did someone's words of encouragement have the opposite effect? It was devastating when you had to cancel plans with your parents. They were always optimistic and hopeful. When we did see each other, they talked about everything else except your health. They maintained their positive attitude and always respected our feelings. They knew what was going on, but all they wanted was to love their son and cherish every moment.

It was also critical that we maintained a strong support system and surrounded ourselves with positive people. There wasn't room for any additional negative energy. I compared us to batteries that were constantly being worn down. We needed people to charge our personal batteries and give us energy when we were running low. We never gave up or allowed ourselves to have the pity party for too long. We learned to handle one setback at a time. We went forward together hoping tomorrow would be better as we went with the flow of the disease. We thought about what we could do and not about what we couldn't. We let go of everything and accepted the fact that we couldn't control the lab screw-ups, doctors, hospitals, drugs, or test results. We accepted whatever happened because it was the way it was supposed to be. "We chose how we were going to handle our choices."

The word NO gave new meaning to my life, when I finally confronted my feelings about rejection, denial, disappointment, and frustration. Once I let go and accepted this challenging time with their emotional overtones as a part of life, it became easier for me to keep up a positive attitude. We did everything we could to give you quality of life and maintain your dignity. We were afraid to be optimistic, but we were more afraid to be afraid. You were able to maintain your remarkable attitude, because you continued to love life and live it to the fullest. Your positive attitude about life was my life.

18 Taking Care of Myself

"You must take care before you give care."

Dear Jeff,

What does the word "caregiving" mean to you? The dictionary says it means watchful, attentive, looked after, and held dear. For me, caregiving is every one of those things and more. Can you give care for an hour or a day? Can it be given weekly, monthly, or is it forever? "Caregiving is whatever you want for as long as you want." Do you think giving care is a choice or should it be expected? Caregiving is a choice and should be given solely from your heart. Is caregiving a simple task or a difficult chore? Does caregiving have to be planned or can it be done spontaneously? "Caregiving is whatever you want for as long as you want." Do you give care to one person or to many? Is the act of caregiving more for the individual receiving care or for the one giving it? Caregiving should feel right for everyone involved. Are you giving care to someone now? Are you cherishing every moment no matter how difficult they may be? Whether giving care through the good times or the bad, never stop doing it. Nothing is more rewarding, personally satisfying, or more greatly appreciated.

While you are giving your care to someone else, who is taking care of you? During the summer of '92, as you were recovering, I realized giving care and taking care were two very different things. If I was going to be an effective caregiver, I needed to stay healthy and strong. How could I be good for you if I wasn't being good to myself? But, trying to meet my own needs during this time was much more difficult and challenging than I ever thought possible. Taking care of myself now required, not only willingness on my part, but an incredible amount of patience. At times it seemed an impossible task because your illness was both serious and long-term. I did not know how I would be able to meet my own needs during that time.

Throughout our twenty-five years, I tried many different things in an attempt to meet my own needs. When we were first married and lived in Albany, you were studying for your master's degree and I worked full time as a dental hygienist. As a student's wife, I felt it my responsibility to type your two-year master's degree program, including your thesis. It was an amazing undertaking and quite an accomplishment. When I wasn't doing your homework, all I wanted to do was cook. You couldn't get me out of the kitchen. I started collecting a library of cookbooks and every day I surprised you with a new recipe. Cooking was something we did together and our meals were gastronomical feasts. Cooking became my passion and in 1990, I wrote a cookbook and started my publishing company. These two years were difficult physically and emotionally, but they were exciting and rewarding. The harder we worked towards our goals, the greater our satisfaction was when we achieved them.

During our three years in Gainesville, you were working on your doctoral degree. When we first moved there, I wanted to try something challenging. I went out and bought a sewing machine. You came home from school and said, "Why did you buy a sewing machine when you don't sew?" I couldn't sew when I bought it, but one week later the bedrooms had curtains and the tables had cloths. I started sewing twenty-four hours a day and made clothes for friends. Between my cooking and sewing classes, homemaking, and helping you through your degree, I grew individually and as your wife. I took care of myself while giving care to you and our home. By becoming self-sufficient, I established my own identity. I learned how to meet many of my own needs because I wanted to.

In Houston, we built our first home. I became fascinated with roses and wanted to design and landscape the yard. Roses grew all year long and it was an exciting challenge building a rose garden. One day, you came home from work and the backyard was landscaped with seventy-five different varieties of roses. There wasn't one bush that was the same. Our garden was magnificent and we had fresh roses every day on the kitchen table. We traveled extensively and entertained friends and colleagues. I was involved with your counseling practice and business. I had several opportunities to cook professionally, but I declined the offers because I wanted to take piano lessons. I hired a tutor for twice a week lessons, practiced three to four hours a day, and gave recitals during our dinner parties. For weeks, you went off to work hearing the same song, but you always said you liked it. We joined a synagogue and became active in our congregation and the community. Though I matured physically, mentally, emotionally and spiritually in Houston, my life always revolved around you, your career, and being your wife.

When we moved to Boca Raton in 1985, I decided to join a gym. I knew nothing about bodybuilding but that's what I wanted to do. I hired a former Mr. America as my instructor and began weight training three hours a day, seven days a week. The more I exercised, the more empowered I became. It was challenging, rewarding, and exceeded my expectations. Bodybuilding gave me greater confidence in myself and helped me respect people more. In 1990, I wrote and published my cookbook; "Safe Sex Never Tasted So Good" and was autographing books at local bookstores. I joined the Chamber of Commerce, was the guest speaker at community functions, and attended charity events. Susan Lee Mintz had become her own person. I was forty years old, I had a beautiful home, a successful husband, and a future that was exciting and fun. But, no one knew the secret I had been keeping for years. In 1981, I chose celibacy rather than risk my health, when I feared you might become HIV positive. Abstinence not only saved my life, it made me stronger. We still continued to share a loving intimate non-sexual relationship and our friendship continued to grow. My life was balanced and I was totally fulfilled.

I was always attracted to your independence, strength, and confidence. Over the years, I was able to pursue my interests because you weren't demanding or "needy." I had the time to meet my needs. Now, I am frightened and confused, and the only thing that matters is your survival. I don't have the time or the energy to think about myself. I am overwhelmed with matters that have to be taken care of immediately. I have to tell our parents, your business colleagues, and friends. I rush home, grab a quick bite, shower, and hurry back to the hospital. One night while I was sitting holding your hand, a terrifying feeling gripped my body. I was speechless and couldn't move. I felt like I was watching someone else go through this ordeal. Instinctively, I grabbed a piece of paper, a pencil, and started to write. Blinded by my tears, I could barely see the paper as I scribbled my thoughts down. My mind was reeling with facts and figures, names and faces. My hands fought desperately to keep up with the endless stream of emotions and frantic feelings pouring out of me.

I found myself documenting every detail of what I was experiencing in a journal. Whether I was emotionally wiped out, physically exhausted, angry, or afraid, every day I wrote my feelings down. As I read the words back to me, they gave me energy, courage, and hope. We started to incorporate everyday things back into our life once you came home. I was lifting weights again, selling cookbooks, and enjoying my community activities. When you felt well, I went about my routine doing the things I normally did. But, when you were ill, your needs were the only ones that were important. These were the times when every aspect of my life revolved around you. This was also the time when my writing became my therapy. It was through my writing that I remained organized, stuck to schedules, and stayed focused as to what had to be done at the time. Your needs were continuing to increase as the disease progressed. You were becoming more dependent upon me and my needs suffered.

I could never get caught up, because there was always something that had to be done. There was an endless amount of laundry. Our meals were never on schedule, and we didn't know from day to day how you would feel. I was running everywhere picking up groceries, supplies, and medications. The phone rang constantly with deliveries, visits from medical personnel, and appointments that had to be both scheduled and many times cancelled. I wasn't sleeping or eating properly. I wasn't taking care of myself. I was physically, mentally, and emotionally depleted. I was functioning automatically like a robot, pushing myself to exhaustion. When I thought there was nothing else I could do, I grabbed my spiral notebook and started to write about the feelings I was experiencing. No matter how unclear, confused, or uncertain my thoughts, my writing brought me the peace I needed to focus on what was important. I realized I had to take care of myself because you needed me more than ever. I owed it to you, our parents, and myself.

My greatest expectations and needs were fulfilled by your constant support, encouragement, and inspiration. No matter what I wanted to do, you guided and assisted me with your honest opinions, common sense, and never-ending patience. You were never judgmental, jealous, or demanding. You admired the pride I took in myself and the passion I had for life. You complimented and recognized my successes and appreciated me. The most rewarding and satisfying times were when I was both giving and taking care of you. Being your wife, a homemaker, and fulfilling my commitment to our marriage was my ultimate accomplishment. I've spent a lot of time thinking about what I have learned from this tragic experience. Though, there were many frustrating times when I felt my needs weren't being met, I believed if I failed you, I would have failed myself. I took care of myself through my writing and documenting a story about the best twenty-five years of my life. From June 20, 1992, through Aug 17, 1994, my fifteen hand-written journals became my fifteen best friends.

19 Laughing Through the Tears

"As children we giggled spontaneously over everything and endlessly over nothing."

Dear Jeff,

During the most stressful and agonizing times of your illness, I asked myself this question, "What would I do if I was an actress, this was a movie, and I was only playing a role? How would I handle this tragedy and cope with the pain? What would I want my audience to see and feel?" The answer would always be the same. I would want to make you laugh and feel better by turning your sadness into something positive and light-hearted. Wouldn't that be wonderful if we were all actors and actresses playing "let's pretend?" How simple life would be if we could walk away after the scene was over leaving our problems behind. Unfortunately, real life isn't a dress rehearsal and there aren't any understudies for your part. And if laughter is the best medicine, how did you feel after a good laugh? Did you sleep more peacefully? Did it help reduce your stress by making some pretty uncomfortable situations not quite so unpleasant? And how many people over the years did a laugh bring together because it was contagious? You once said "laughing was easy to do and fun to share." I said, "laughter is addicting because it lulls you into a state of euphoria." For me, this feel good feeling helped me handle my worst problems with hope.

I was taught in school that there were five senses. They were the sense of sight, sound, smell, taste, and touch. As I got older, I discovered I possessed two other intensely powerful senses. They both were about choice, letting go of control and acceptance. The sixth sense is called my Common Sense. I think you are either born with this trait or you are not. The seventh sense is the most difficult one to maintain, but it is the most important one of all. It is called A Sense of Humor. Laughter and humor helped us to toughen up as life's setbacks and disappointments kept coming along. The humor managed to keep everything in perspective and it protected us from further pain and suffering. Being able to laugh during these two years kept us together and strengthened our bond. Sometimes the humor got misplaced, but eventually we found it again. And no matter how horrible the situation, for twenty-five years, we managed to keep our seventh sense. For me, these two senses became my best friends helping me when nothing else would. Now, at this crossroads in my life, I've asked for their assistance and support more than ever before.

Since the fifth grade, you always made me laugh with your quick wit and silly comebacks. When Mom heard the laughs coming from my room, she knew we were talking on the phone. We laughed about school, friends, television, and at each other. We liked telling jokes, playing games, and exchanging letters. You always found something humorous to talk about and our friendship was built upon laughter and fun. Your beautiful smile and gentle happy voice made me feel alive. Remembering all the wonderful laughs we've shared has helped me through the first few weeks. Those memories brought back joyful times with happy feelings. But, where is the humor in the possibility of your death and the suffering everyone is enduring? How can I find anything to laugh about now? I was brought to tears when you smiled at me in the hospital. How could one smile reaffirm that you were back in my life? It took a while before we laughed again, but we always managed to give each other a whole lot of smiles.

I remember the first time we really laughed again. You went into the hospital on June 20th, weighing 165 pounds and came home two weeks later weighing 145 pounds. Because I loved to cook, we assumed you would put the twenty pounds back on quickly. We were sadly mistaken. The adjustment to our new life was much more difficult than we had imagined. You forced yourself to eat and we weren't handling the food and medication issue well. One of your drugs had to be taken at breakfast with fatty foods. I went into the kitchen, looked at these 3 giant pills, and out of sheer frustration yelled, "To hell with this." I found a sterling silver tray, placed a red linen napkin in the center, and jammed the horse pills into the middle of a Snickers candy bar. I changed into a nightgown and we pretended we were dining in Paris, France. We were hysterical and decided to make a game out of it. You picked out the cities and I looked for the most delicious fattening foods that matched. For several weeks, breakfast was served at 9:00AM and surprise sugar and pills were the entrée. You enjoyed taking your medications, gained back the weight, and got stronger. Whenever we saw a candy bar, we giggled.

You would say, "Get out the drugs, I'm going to have a feast." On one of our cruises we went to a midnight dessert buffet. We fell all over ourselves laughing as we ran back to the room, gathered up your pills, and imagined all the different ways you could take your drugs on this vacation.

As your appetite increased and you wanted to eat, it was your chronic diarrhea that made it difficult for you to gain weight. Every morning you went into the bathroom, weighed yourself, and came out saying, "The big guy is holding his own." What made this funny was that you put on your boxer shorts, leaped into the room, and started doing bodybuilding poses. We played old disco music and you danced. I would close my eyes and when I opened them you would be in another pose. Tears streamed down our cheeks as we howled with laughter. Another time you started to juice because you wanted to build up your immune system. We bought an industrial strength juicer and every day you made a twelve-ounce glass of carrot juice. The orange pigment caused your skin, urine, and stools to change color. One morning, you came flying out of the bathroom yelling, "I think I just pooped a whole carrot. My entire stool is orange and it's huge." I went in and it looked exactly like a carrot.

We were hysterical thinking about the assortment of colors your stools could be. I said, "What would you eat to make a rainbow?" Going to the bathroom became something we could laugh about.

Planning meals was very difficult and dinners became stressful and unpredictable at times. We never knew if you would be well enough to eat. One night you wanted lamb chops with lemon, garlic, and butter. Your appetite was great and the meal was delicious. As we relaxed after the meal, without warning your face turned green. You said, "I'm going to throw up." You never made it to the bathroom. You heaved and hurled chunks of lamb everywhere. I yelled, "You're having a f….ing exorcism like Linda Blair in the movie." You almost choked on your own vomit, you laughed so hard. Though it was a horrible experience, we laughed about it for a long time.

One night after your second bout with pneumonia, you wanted Chinese buffet for dinner. You were weak and your appetite was terrible. But, I was so excited because you wanted to eat. You also wanted a drink. Usually, I would have been afraid that the combination of drugs and alcohol would be harmful. But that night, I didn't care about anything. I wanted to enjoy watching you eat. We ordered a drink and were feeling great. You went to get your food but came back with an empty plate. I asked you if there was something wrong. You said you wanted Italian food instead. We excused ourselves and left. We got to the other restaurant and you ordered another drink. Now I was upset and said, "What the hell are you doing?" You said, "I have AIDS, Susan. Do you think a drink is going to kill me?" The waiter came over and you ordered dinner. When he brought your dinner out, you smelled it and said, "I'm going to throw up." The waiter got upset because he thought it was something he had done. I said, "You are not the problem. My husband hasn't been feeling well." You turned that horrible shade of green again and threw up on the waiter. The manager ran over apologizing about everything. They were convinced we were going to sue them, but I assured them we hadn't eaten anything. He begged us to come back for dinner and it would be on him. We almost wet our pants laughing when he said dinner would literally be on the house. On the way home, you said, "I should go out to dinner every night. What a way to get a free meal." When we got into bed, we were still chuckling about our dining experience.

Your parents moved closer and lived in an assisted living facility down the street. Your mother's visits were carefully supervised because she was suffering with Alzheimer 's disease, and her erratic behavior disturbed you. I usually took her for a walk, enabling you and Dad to spend some quality time together. One day, you said you were tired of staying in bed and wanted to visit with them in the den. By now, you weren't able to control your bodily functions and were wearing a diaper. You took the walker and proceeded down the hall. Your parents followed single file behind you. I stopped, stood back, and observed the site before me. You were shuffling, pushing your walker, and your diaper was rustling. Dad was shuffling close behind you, and your mother was shuffling and rustling in her diaper. It was a perfectly choreographed production. I excused myself because I was emotionally out of control and beginning to get hysterical. How could this be my life? I was forty-seven years old, watching the three people I love become strangers. They were my family, yet I barely recognized them. All of a sudden, the crying turned into uncontrollable laughter and I wet my pants. Now, I was the one who needed the diaper. I thought of the different songs and phrases that went with rustling diapers. Songs like "shake, rattle, and tootsie roll," "rustling diapers in the wind," "don't let it poop on my parade." If you all had pooped at the same time, I'd never be able to clean up the mess.

So, when nothing seems right and you don't know what else to do, remember your Seventh Sense. It will get you through the worst of times and it's all yours. No one can take it away from you. We chose to laugh a lot during our twenty-five years. We laughed at our challenges, the obstacles, and even the frightening aspects of your mortality. You made me laugh when I cried for you, and I made you laugh when you were afraid. We brought out the best in each other and the laughter was certainly the best. Sometimes I laugh through my tears because I miss you. But, now I am smiling, my darling Jeffrey. Can you see it?

20 I was Angry and Hated Myself

> "We were growing together while we were growing apart."

Dear Jeff,

What did I really want out of life? Did you know I had to go through a difficult and troubled childhood, a roller coaster tumultuous marriage, and a battle with a deadly disease for me to finally be able to answer that question? And what do you think my answer finally was? "I got out of it exactly what I wanted to." My only regret is that I wish it hadn't taken me so long to realize how unnecessarily cruel I was to myself, and how much valuable time and energy I wasted as I vented my frustration and anger on the ones I loved. In the past, whenever someone asked me if I was happy, I sarcastically responded, "Yes, when I'm eating chocolate ice cream or listening to music." I never could answer that question comfortably without hesitating because I didn't understand what happiness was all about. However, I was quite familiar with the subject of unhappiness having dealt with this feeling throughout much of my life.

As a young child, I was stubborn, difficult, and moody. As a teenager, whenever I got frustrated I became angry, volatile and mean. If I didn't get my way, I was argumentative, resisted authority, and antagonistic. I loved being challenged and lost interest in things quickly. I found it easy for me to manipulate and overpower people. And at eighteen years of age, I was searching for the perfect parents, the perfect life, and the perfect husband. I wanted a life that was glamorous, exciting, and that life didn't exist in Troy, New York. These were the things I thought I wanted out of life because that would make me happy. Nothing was going to stop me from going after what I wanted. Unfortunately, the more I searched for perfection in a less than perfect world, the more my frustration and hostility grew. My quest was doing me more harm than good, but I continued to blame everyone else for my problems. I was establishing a self-destructive pattern of behavior that I eventually brought into our marriage. And those were some of my good qualities.

There was one person who really understood and accepted me. He thought I was unique and fun because I made him laugh. That boy was Jeffrey A. Mintz. You were gentle, sweet, even tempered and a great listener. If the saying "opposites attract" is true, we were a perfect example of the slogan's meaning. Our personalities complemented and balanced each other making us a powerful team. Many times I said, "our friendship was perfect, but the marriage was hell." In 1969, I was twenty-two years old, immature, unhappy and angry about my pregnancy and miscarriage. I was having a difficult time adjusting to my marriage and a new life. I blamed you for my unhappiness and I became verbally abusive. I attacked you with cold cruel comments like, "I know you didn't want to marry me. You had to because it was the right thing to do. I hate being a dental hygienist and a student's wife. You are always studying. We're on a budget. I'm sick of typing your work." When I didn't feel well, I looked for any reason to lash out at you. I wanted you to hurt as badly as I did. When you confessed about your bisexuality, my resentment towards you increased. Wherever we moved, I carried my anger and hostility along with me. Through your master's degree in Albany, your doctorate in Gainesville, and your counseling practice in Houston, our horrible fighting continued. We were growing together while growing apart.

No matter how difficult our marriage became, I was able to convince myself that all relationships have their share of problems. I could rationalize any situation until it satisfied my needs. Together, we were a team. We looked good together, had fun, shared the same goals, and cared about each other. I always managed to get the good things to outweigh the bad. But, your bisexuality hurt me the most, because I didn't trust you anymore. Your nights out with your lovers were destroying me. My frustration and rage was consuming me and I wanted to hurt you with vicious, heartless words. As the arguments intensified, I'd scream at you, "Why did you marry me? Why do you stay with me? Why don't you get out? You're the one who is gay. Just get out." On several different occasions you did walk out, but you always came back. You came back because you knew how difficult it was for me to deal with your lifestyle and sexuality. And you also knew I loved you and I knew you loved me.

The eleven years we lived in Houston were bittersweet, as we continued to bring out the best and the worst in each other. We knew we shouldn't be together, but we didn't want to be apart. Our marriage had become a complicated co-dependent relationship based upon deception, dishonesty, and distrust. We were enmeshed in each other lives, caught up in a catch-22. You were leading a secretive double life and were having numerous sexual relationships with different men. However, you were an established doctor with a successful counseling practice and management company. We were active members in our synagogue and the community. I wasn't working any longer and my life as a beautiful doctor's wife appeared perfect. When I put on my makeup and flashed that million-dollar smile, no one would ever doubt the lies and half-truths I told. In an attempt to cover up my anger and growing resentment towards you and my life, I told off-color sexual jokes, became brutally sarcastic, and enjoyed making cutting wisecracks.

When I first heard about AIDS in 1981, I knew someday you would need me more than ever. For me now, it didn't matter how difficult or agonizing my marriage might become. I had to accept your homosexual affairs under any condition. However, I set one condition up for myself. I made a decision to abstain from having a sexual relationship with you in order to protect myself from possible HIV infection. When we moved to Boca Raton in 1985, I thought there was a chance you might change, since most of your lovers in Houston had died or were HIV positive. Though you knew the AIDS epidemic had become a frightening and real possibility in our life, you were whom you were and you were never going to change.

When you went out of town on business, it was understood that you were having sex with different men. Alone in my bed at night, I would say over and over again, "Jeff, you must be careful. You know you are at risk. You were promiscuous for years. Why are you killing yourself?" I was desperately afraid, but couldn't tell anyone that my husband was gay and could possibly get AIDS. I'd kept secrets about our marriage, my pregnancy, and the miscarriage, but this secret was the most frightening one because I feared for my husband's life. I continued to respect your wishes to keep your secret and our private life private, but I desperately needed to tell someone the truth. All my years of denial and rationalizing had finally caught up with me, and the lies had eaten at me like a cancer. I was becoming despondent, depressed, and I was on the verge of collapse. I wanted to scream, "I'm not who you think I am. The person you see is someone else. I can't keep these secrets inside me any longer."

On June 19th, 1992, along with your illness came the truth about our life together. Family, friends, and colleagues had to be told that you had AIDS. We had to be honest with everyone about everything for the first time, because we would not be able to keep our secrets any longer. Your illness forced us to confront our worst fears and address the issues we were afraid to talk about before. The time had finally come for me to purge twenty-three years of deception and lies. The disease had given me permission to let go and allow my healing process to begin. I had brought many of my previous deep-seated frustrations and unresolved personal conflicts into the relationship. I didn't like myself, but I didn't know any other way to handle my frustrations. It was easier to blame you for my problems, and I looked for any excuse to avoid facing the truth about myself. Now, I had come face to face with my past and realized that it was my own inadequacies and weaknesses I didn't like. Blaming you for getting ill or hating your sexual partners and your bisexuality would not change anything.

The problems in our marriage, the issues of bisexuality, and now the pressures of a serious illness made us continue to say things and respond to situations like never before. The challenges of this difficult time made the good things between us better and the bad things worse. The frustration and fear we felt now brought out both our strengths and our weaknesses. But, AIDS was the source of our pain, and we couldn't allow the disease to destroy our relationship. We learned to take our frustrations out on the disease and not each other. We accepted the fact that a long-term illness under these conditions would be overwhelming for both of us. The demands during this time were going to be more than we ever expected. I remember saying to you one day, "If life isn't perfect, why do we have to be?" We strengthened our bond in marriage and in friendship because we were finally open and honest about our life.

Now, I am much kinder to myself and understand that blaming life for my problems didn't accomplish anything. I had to grow up and become responsible for my actions. I buried my anger, rage, guilt, and blame along with you. I became a woman I could respect and the person you trusted with your life.

There were many times after you died when I asked myself the same questions I'd asked of you for twenty-five years. "Why did I stay with you? Why didn't I have the courage to get out? Why couldn't I have had the love I'd always wanted? Why was I weak?" My answers were always the same as yours. I never left because I loved you. We made our marriage what we wanted it to be. "Till death do us part" from a deadly disease would be the only way our passionate twenty-five-year bond would end.

21 Coping with Frustration and Fear

"My emotional foundation is on the verge of collapse. The simplest tasks have now become difficult complex chores."

July 1994

Dear Jeff,

I've been writing in my journal a lot more often these days. My writing has become both my therapy and my best friend. It brings me comfort, support, and is helping me to stay focused. The never-ending demands of your illness are more than I ever imagined. My mind races continuously with horrible nightmarish thoughts and I am exhausted from thinking about the frightening "what if" questions that do not have any answers. I haven't slept through the night in months and must force myself to eat. I am not sticking to schedules, managing to stay caught up, or using my time effectively. It's been months since we've enjoyed a few days without a crisis.

I am not meeting my own personal needs and my emotions are raging out of control. I am blowing the smallest things out of proportion, my coping mechanism is overloaded, and I do not know when I will explode. I find myself withdrawn and depressed one moment and responding aggressively the next. I am anxious, uncertain, and fearful that I will react instinctively and make hasty decisions that will be wrong or cause you further suffering. My reactions, attitude, and mood swings are unpredictable because I am frustrated and afraid. I do not think I will ever have the energy or desire to have fun again.

Over the years, we faced many difficult situations and went through some pretty rough times. But, we were able to meet our challenges because we were very capable and competent in making decisions. We were frustrated due to the uncertainty of our decisions and frightened because of the unknown outcome. However, our fears and frustrations vanished once we dealt with the problem and moved on. But, the challenges and obstacles we faced before were nothing compared to the ones we were dealing with now. I am terrified everyday of what might or might not happen and frustrated about why something did or did not.

For two years, I have lived in a perpetual state of fear and the constant stress and strain has taken its toll on my physical, mental, and emotional well-being. The tension I am under every day is agonizingly painful. I am finding it more difficult to adjust to the sudden unexpected changes happening to you. My ability to cope and my emotional stability is being influenced and determined by everything from the weather, money issues, traffic delays, or cancelled doctor's appointments. And timing, as well as fear and frustration, has made simple everyday routine situations more complicated and sometimes dangerous. Timing is the number one factor determining whether the uncertainty and instability of a situation will be either tolerable or unbearable. Timing has turned the simple into difficult and made the difficult monumental.

As your wife, caregiver, and friend, I was on call twenty-four hours a day. I used to say that, "when you were all right, so was I," because it was nearly impossible to take care of you and myself at the same time. However, your three hospital stays with pneumonia were the most difficult and stressful times

I faced. What made them even more frightening was that their uncertain outcomes could possibly be tragic ones. When I was home alone, I went about my work, handled my responsibilities, and functioned. I performed like a robot because everything I thought about or did revolved around you in the hospital. I could not eat or sleep because I was running back and forth at all hours of the day and night. I yelled at everyone and constantly cried. I couldn't make the simplest decisions about stupid things like what I should wear. Should I stay over with you? Should I bring your parents? I could not handle the dozens of unanswered "should I" questions because simple wasn't simple any longer.

Our life had been permanently changed with your diagnosis. You weren't having your tonsils out. You were dying from AIDS. How could anything ever be simple again? Do you remember the first time I said, "Jeff, nothing is ever going to be simple again?" It was the night we had the flat tire and you needed to get to the hospital. Though flat tires had inconvenienced us before you took ill, they were not life threatening experiences. We once missed a flight to Europe. Another time we were late for a wedding. And on our honeymoon in Spain, a tire blew in the middle of a vicious thunderstorm and we went spinning around. But, I never imagined something as simple and routine as a flat tire could cause such panic and fear. It was a cool spring evening in April 1993. You had been coughing and spiking dangerously high fevers for several days. The x-ray revealed that your pneumonia had returned. You were scheduled to go into the hospital the following day for a two-week intravenous treatment.

That night, your fever spiked to 104.5 degrees. You were convulsing and delusional. I couldn't get you cooled down. I called our doctor telling him you were gravely ill and needed immediate medical treatment. He said he would meet us at the hospital emergency room. I managed to get you dressed and literally carried you into the elevator and to the car. I couldn't get the door open so I propped you up against the trunk. I started the car, came around and got you, and as I backed the car out, we heard a rocking noise and the car was shaking. It was 1:00 AM, the night was chilly. There we were with a flat, and our other car was being serviced. I wrapped you in a blanket and made you lie down in the back seat. Adrenaline surged through my body and I thought my heart would leap from my chest. For a brief moment, I panicked fearing for your life. I ran upstairs and called 911. Within minutes, the ambulance arrived and took you to the hospital. For me, a simple flat tire became a frighteningly dangerous situation.

Before you took ill, I never thought about the expression, "do you live to eat or eat to live?" For twenty-five years, we shared a passion for food. We enjoyed cooking and eating together more than anything else we did. You had an incredible appetite, ate everything I made, and usually asked for seconds. We planned many meals completely around a new cuisine with foods we had never tried before. It was great fun creating new and exciting recipes from different countries. We made our dinners fantastic adventures that were incredibly delicious. You loved coming home to "guess what's cooking in Susan's kitchen night."

But, you aren't eating for fun any longer. You are eating to stay alive. It didn't matter whether it was a cracker, a cookie, a piece of bread, or a scoop of ice cream; all I wanted you to do was eat. In January 1994, you developed your third bout of pneumonia. You continued to lose a tremendous amount of weight and by April 1994, your condition had taken a critical turn for the worst. Your immune system was seriously compromised and you were symptomatic with other medical conditions. One day out of sheer terror, I called the doctor. I was frantic. I told him if you didn't get your appetite back soon, it was going to be too late. He put you on supplements, appetite stimulants, and fortified drinks. I made you protein shakes, fresh fruit drinks, made your favorite foods, and did middle of the night food runs. By July, nothing we tried helped. You didn't have enough energy to eat any longer.

In twenty-five years, I never remember hearing you raise your voice to your parents. You adored each other and talked about everything. By July, we knew I needed help with your care. The time had come for Hospice to assist us both. You couldn't live like this any longer. Your parents came over for their visit and you told them about your decision. They continued to visit daily for several weeks, but their time spent with you gradually became shorter because you tired easily. Your visits with Dad were never a problem, but Mom's Alzheimer's disease caused her to make repetitious remarks and meaningless outbursts. These became increasingly frustrating and exhausting. As your condition worsened, your patience with her became less until one day you couldn't take it any

.. Mom started to ramble on and though barely able to speak, you looked at me and said, "Please get her out of here. I cannot listen to this anymore." Dad and I knew how much you loved your mother. But it was horribly painful and saddening to hear you tell your mom to leave the room. After that incident, I continued to take Mom to see you, but immediately took her out of the apartment.

Another incident made me brutally aware of how overwhelming and exhausting a long term life threatening illness can be. By June, you were not able to take care of yourself and were becoming completely dependent on me. I developed a bronchial infection, a 102-degree fever, and could barely get out of bed. I felt like every nerve in my body was on fire. For days, I hadn't been able to sleep because you were up every night with a fever and coughing. My doctor said he would call me in an antibiotic. I flew out of the house leaving you alone. When I got to the pharmacy, my prescription wasn't ready. I was told my doctor hadn't called it in yet. It was a holiday weekend. The office was closed, and he'd gone out of town. It took two hours for another doctor to call the script in. I was screaming at the pharmacist and crying hysterically at the same time. I was emotionally out of control and took my rage and frustration out on an innocent person. I reacted this way because I was frustrated and desperately afraid for you.

Over the years, a few of our decisions didn't turn out the way we hoped they would, but we became more flexible as we compromised and adjusted to the setbacks and disappointments. After you were diagnosed, however, we lived by a different set of rules and our compromises now weren't so easy to do. We faced frightening issues that didn't allow us any choices. Whether it was our emotional stability or the disease's progress, our life became one unpredictable chaotic conflict and nothing would ever be stable, normal, or routine again. And alongside us every step of the way were our two emotional components of fear and frustration. Life was simple until it became complicated.

22 What to do when nothing is Working

"You taught me to believe that the true meaning of life was our desire for life."

July 11, 1994

Dear Jeff,

My mother turned eighty-three years old today. She's been through many ups and downs in her long life and she still is going strong. You, my love, are forty-seven years old and you will not live to see summer's end. You really did try everything imaginable as you battled for two years to survive this illness. It was your incredible will to live that was your strongest drive. One of the many reasons why your will to live was so powerful was because it was your nature to love life and live it to the fullest. Another reason was because you would never have given up on anything you wanted or believed in. You would never have quit and walked away from something just because it got rough and things weren't working out. Throughout your life, it was your will to live that enabled you to endure the most difficult and challenging times. It was your never give up attitude that continued making you believe you could beat the odds. Even now in your final days, you still possess that remarkable will to live, but you do not have the energy to continue the fight. Though you do not want to give up, you can't go on any longer. Your suffering has become impossible to bear.

In June, we finally heard your doctor's words telling you there was nothing else he could do. Our first reactions of shock and disbelief gave way to panic and terror. The dreaded reality of this time had come, but I couldn't accept it. It was too painful to believe you were going to die after you fought so long and so hard to live. I continued calling your doctors frantically pleading with them to find one more drug, treatment, or procedure that could help you. I was begging them, "Why can't any of you find something else that will work? Please do not let him die." But, my pleas and prayers for help went unanswered this time. The doctors could not find anything else in their little black bags that would save your life. How could I deal with the horrible truth that your treatments weren't working any longer and there's nothing left that anyone can do? It is impossible to explain the feelings of helplessness and hopelessness I experienced at this time. I was petrified and terrified. I have never felt this kind of desperation and futility before. I could not let you go. I was not ready to say good bye.

When you were diagnosed in 1992, the AIDS virus had only been discovered ten years before. We hoped for that lifesaving cure we heard was just around the corner. We were optimistic and encouraged because the government was releasing more revenues for research and development. The insurance companies were going to make more alternative treatments accessible and affordable. But, we were walking a fine line as we balanced our hope for a future with the deadly reality of time. We knew there weren't going to be any vaccines or cures coming along in the immediate future. There also weren't many long-term studies available, because most AIDS patients died shortly after they became ill or within a couple of years. Much of the documented medical information and clinical reports only reinforced the frightening facts we already knew. You were going to have to try many powerful drugs with potentially lethal side effects and endure long uncomfortable procedures throughout the course of the disease. We were taking a gamble on everything you tried, but we didn't have a choice. As soon as a drug or treatment was FDA approved, you had access to it. We focused on whatever we needed to do now in order to keep you alive, and we could continue to believe that you would never run out of options.

In June 1992, when you entered the hospital with pneumonia, the doctors decided to put you on a drug that was proven to be highly successful in treating this strain of AIDS bacteria. You were going to be in the hospital for an indefinite period of time and immediately started on a two week/four times a day intravenous treatment. Your doctors believed you would come through this crisis because the clinical data and statistics supported their opinions. It was their words of encouragement and support that helped us remain positive during those two weeks. After you completed the recommended course of treatment, the pneumonia was gone, and you were well enough to leave the hospital. You continued doing twice-weekly inhalations treatments at home. Though you suffered some terrible side effects from these treatments and had difficulty with several other medications, for nine months the pneumonia did not come back. This was our honeymoon period with the disease and during this time we had hope about everything. We half-heartedly believed you might beat the odds.

The most frustrating thing we dealt with during these two years was the fact that no matter how hard you tried, you never regained your strength or got back to the same level you were before you became ill. When the pneumonia did come back nine months later, we were devastated. This was the worst setback we had experienced so far. You reentered the hospital for another two-week course of intravenous antibiotics. But, your immune system was weaker than before the first bout and the treatments had taken a terrible toll on your health in general. When you came home this time, it was even more difficult for you to put the weight back on and you had much less energy. Our doctor said the home inhalation treatments weren't going to work any longer. He put you on several newly approved AIDS medications but you couldn't tolerate their side effects. However, we still continued to believe something else could be done. When the pneumonia came back for the third time in January 1994, even the hospital intravenous treatments were not effective. Your oral medications would not prevent recurrent infections and the massive amounts of anti-viral drugs you were taking to boost your immune system weren't helping either.

Your white blood cell count was critically low causing you to become highly susceptible to dozens of life-threatening infections. Your hemoglobin and red blood cell counts had been nearly destroyed by the disease and the medications, and you had to go into the hospital for a series of blood transfusions. You went in at 9:00AM and when I brought you home at 4:00PM, you developed a case of hiccups that lasted for six weeks. Nothing you tried would get rid of them. You were given protein injections three times a week and several other newly released antibiotics. You were doing Chinese herbs, juicing, acupuncture, ozone therapy, meditation, and megavitamin injections. We continued to believe there would be something else for us to try. But, your time was running out and you were getting weaker and weaker. We were terrified because you were running out of options. There was a sense of urgency and panic setting in that we had not experienced before. This was the oppressing and overpowering realization that you were going to die.

For two years, we put our faith in the power of our love and our trust in the expert medical advice of our doctors. We read dozens of books, magazines, and newspaper articles about experimental new treatments and unconventional therapies. We watched videos and listened to tapes for hours in an attempt to learn more about AIDS. We thought maybe our doctors missed something, anything, and we could find it ourselves. We would not allow each other to give up. We met up with a lot of roadblocks and had to take a few detours, but we were never at a dead end. We wanted to continue to hear words like "encouraging" and "promising." We pleaded with the doctors to tell us anything that might make a difference. We appealed to everyone to please help us find one more thing that could save your life. But, you had run out of time and there wasn't anything left to try. You didn't want to give up, but your fight had been slowly and cruelly drained from you. You wanted to live, but you were too tired now. I wanted you to stay with me just a little longer, but I didn't want to see you suffer any more. This was an excruciating time for us because you had done everything possible to stay alive and all the pleading, begging, crying, and praying in the world would not change the outcome.

By July, all we had left was our hope for a miracle. Nothing could ever possibly compare to the empty feeling in our heart when we finally acknowledged that it was over.

You had some quality times with an abundance of hope, dozens of choices, and lots of plans for the future. You were able to manage the disease effectively for a while with the help of the doctors and the newest medications. Many times you responded favorably to these drugs and the procedures. You constantly experimented with conventional medical treatments as well as controversial alternative ones. We didn't deceive ourselves for one moment by thinking we had a guarantee that anything we did would work. We never expected to hear the words 100 percent. But, what we needed to hear were the constant words of encouragement and reassurance that you had a chance and that there was another option.

Eventually, though you did everything you could, you went from having many choices and options to having none at all. The long-term effects of the illness finally destroyed your physical, mental, emotional, and spiritual well-being and the constant fears and frustrations created additional chaos and turmoil. Our hopes and dreams had finally given way to failure, frustration, and fear. We didn't want to give up, but we had to. This illness was like the lottery. Your chances of losing were far greater than winning. We were playing Russian roulette with a gun that was fully loaded. Your instinct to survive and your desire for life kept us believing tomorrow would be better. Your courage, strength, and will to live gave me the energy and faith to fight till the end with you. You never gave up hope or lost your will to live. You were the bravest man I have ever known.

"For me, love was to sacrifice everything."

"There was a big difference between staying alive and being alive."

Dear Jeff,

The writing in my journal not only documents your illness, it has given me a reason to live. I have now completed my sixth journal. The seventh one begins with the words, "I know that your death is near." Please understand that I did the best I could, but I feel that it wasn't enough. I am at the most frightening turning point in my life and I am not handling your illness well. I am not sure of what decisions to make, what things will work, or whom I should trust. I am terribly sorry about the vicious fight we had the other day. I completely lost it and have never felt this emotionally out of control. I stood before you screaming, "You killed yourself. I gave you my heart, my image, my life. I was your cover. You looked straight when we were together. You took ᴛᴏm me, you took from everyone, and now you are suffering the consequences." As I ripped up the thousands of dollars of drug receipts and threw them over the balcony into the bushes, I was yelling hysterically, "Here is your AIDS scattered all over the yard, just like you have torn apart my life into meaningless shreds." You crawled back into bed and quietly said, "Susan, you need help. You are not coping with this and you are no good for me. It is only going to get worse."

You woke up later that evening coughing violently because the pneumonia had returned again. I could barely understand your whispered words as you said, "Please forgive me. I love you so, but I don't know how to handle this either. I am afraid." We held each other as if it was for the last time. We felt closer at that moment than we had in two years. We both knew why this argument happened. The horrifying end was in sight and letting go was going to be the most difficult thing we would have to do. Every day, I watched your withered body continue to waste away. I felt your anguish, as you were slowly letting go of your life. You are so very frail and frightened. You are slipping away before my eyes and I cannot do anything about it. I am tired of hoping, giving, and being in pain. I am angry and fearful, but I feel helpless and hopeless. My feelings of failure and defeat only intensify the rage and frustration I am experiencing now. I do not want to think, speak, or feel. I want to forget.

How many times have I wished I could die along with you? I am begging for a sign telling me that one day I will be all right again. I need something to give me the strength and courage to continue on. Though I write the words "letting go" down on paper, I do not feel this way in my heart. I can tell myself I must let you go, but I do not believe the words I say. How do I let go of the man I have loved since I was eleven years old and how do I tell my heart to say good bye forever?

There is a monumental difference between staying alive and being alive. You are alive but you are not living. You are now unable to take care of yourself and have become totally dependent upon me. You weigh 120 pounds and have had chronic diarrhea for three weeks. You are coughing so intensely that it causes you to throw up. Your medications are endless and you have gotten too weak to take some of them. The constant fevers have affected your brilliant mind. You have a blank look on your face and forget things easily. You cannot focus. You feel dizzy, and have fainted because you will not eat. You can barely stay awake, don't have the energy to shower, and can hardly brush your once beautiful white teeth. You can't remember nor understand most of the things going on around you. However, you maintained your control over the most important and powerful issue of them all. How you wanted to live out the rest of your life.

On July 8th, you called your doctor and said, "I am the patient and I am not going back into the hospital again. I'm in charge of what I will or will not do from now on. The final weeks of my life will be on my own terms. I will allow people to help us with my care and we will set the house up so I can die at home. That is the way it will be." I knew then you did not want to live any longer, but I couldn't accept it and didn't have the courage to bring it up. You didn't have the energy to eat and you wanted to sleep all the time. I had to brush your teeth, wash your hair, clean your nails, and shave and bathe you in bed. It was a tragedy for you to watch your beautiful body deteriorate. The day came when you gave me a look that told me everything I needed to know. With unspoken words and a glance I shall never forget, I knew you were ready to accept your death. You had given yourself permission to die. No words could express the intensity of the moment we shared. We knew without saying anything what we had to do and what was going to happen.

For twenty-five years, we enjoyed a life that was private and a relationship that was personal and intimate. We made our homes warm and inviting and there was always the fragrance of delicious foods lingering in the air. The sounds of good conversation, music, and laughter filled the rooms when we entertained family and friends. With great sadness, we had to let go of the life we once loved in order for you to have some quality of life now. We had to allow the outside world into ours. We had become prisoners trapped inside our home and our captor was the disease that had destroyed our lives. Every day we became more dependent upon the nurses, the medical deliveries, and the lab technicians. We signed dozens of consent forms, requests, and legal documents. And with every signature, we relinquished a little more of our control. We were "letting go" of our cherished privacy, freedom, and independence.

Our home became a hospital setting with supplies and drugs everywhere. There were people in and out, but they were not our friends bringing laughter and good cheer. They were strangers taking care of you and assisting me. We never had to trust many people before because we always had each other. But, now letting go meant trusting everyone and that was something very difficult for us to do. You had to let go of your pride as others assisted you and pitied you at the same time. Letting go now meant waiting for death even though you were still alive. Letting go meant suffering and heartache for your parents. Letting go meant giving up your business, your love for travel and adventure, your passion for food, and everything fun you enjoyed.

Letting go was also difficult because it meant saying our final good-byes. Letting go meant being alone and I didn't want to live without you. Letting go meant you would not be there to eat dinner with me. Letting go meant I wouldn't be watching movies or walking on the beach with you any longer. Letting go meant you would not be there to hold me when I desperately needed to be held. Though I had buried you a hundred times in my mind, I could not stop my heart from loving and wanting you. How could I say good-bye to my best friend? Letting go meant missing you. Oh, how I will miss you. You were letting go of your life while I was letting go of everything I had ever loved. And finally, I had to let go of the anger I was feeling towards you and this disease. I had to stop hating you for getting ill. I had to stop hating myself for staying with you. I had to let go of the hate I had for my life because living it was more painful than I had been willing to admit. I had to let go of the anger and hate or I would not have been able to stay with you through this. I looked in the mirror and said, "Susan, give yourself permission to let go. You have some choices left. Everything hasn't been taken from you. Allow yourself to give it up." Letting go now had become allowing myself to let go. I knew now I could handle the last few weeks of my life with you.

Changing my perspective did not make my loss any easier, but it did enable me to go on afterwards with great peace of mind and a renewed sense of purpose. Allowing myself permission to let go helped cleanse, heal, and strengthen my broken heart. As I look back over our years together, I know we both liked being in control. But, what did we want to be in control of? We had choices and made decisions, but we did not have control. Feeling in control was both deceptive and elusive, because it was a feeling that could be lost in seconds. I found out the more I fought to stay in control, the harder it would be for me to let go. Letting go was part of the dying process and denying the outcome would not have prevented it.

I was stupid enough to think it would be easier to let go if I used less frightening words like to release, to liberate, or to free from blame. But, this was a futile ridiculous attempt to ease my suffering, because the process of letting go wasn't about words. Letting go was about feelings that involved the most painful experience of my life. Letting go was about sorrow and tragedy because I'd have to accept the finality of our life together. Letting go was impossible for me because I couldn't let this disease force me into letting go of you and the wonderful life we made for each other. The only way I would be able to handle this time was to completely relinquish all control and give myself permission to let go. If I could allow myself to do this and let go, I would be able to accept your death. I had to give myself a choice. On August 17, 1994, I said my ultimate goodbye as I watched you let go of your life. There was one final thing we never did let go of, and that was our need to need each other even during the final days of your life. And the one thing I will never have to let go of are my beautiful memories of a wonderful man who gave me the best and worst years of my life. I'll never let go of my love for you.

24 *Saying GoodBye*

"We've shared a lifetime and lifeline of love."

"It wasn't until after you died that I would understand the power of this organization and the importance of its concept in my life."

August 3, 1994

Dear Jeff,

The past few weeks have gone by so slowly, yet somehow they vanished in an instant. I crawled into bed next to you and held your tired body in my arms. Your empty darkly circled eyes stared through me. I said, "You wanted to starve yourself to death, didn't you? You knew you wanted to die and this was the way you could do it. I can still see us sitting at the kitchen table. Your one look said it all. Your eyes told me what you wanted next. I felt the same way, my love, but it was your decision to make. My poor baby. You couldn't go through any more suffering. You wanted to take control again of your life." You whispered, "Yes. Anything would be better than living like this." I said, "Why didn't you admit what you wanted to do? Your parents and friends love you. Everyone would have understood and respected your wishes." I leaned closer and you said, "As long as you knew what I wanted, that was all I cared about. You were the one who would see me through this. You've always been my Godsend." You smiled your beautiful smile and winked your special wink. Oh, my darling love, I knew you wouldn't admit it to anyone but me. As warm gentle tears ran down my cheeks, you fell peacefully asleep in my arms. My heart ached for this man I adored and would lose just fourteen days later.

I must go back to July 2nd. I want to sleep on the floor next to you, so I picked up a foam mattress for the side of the bed. You sleep most of the time, but I have to change your diaper and turn you every few hours. Your needs are simple and few, but they continue twenty-four-hours a day. It's 8:30 PM and I ran out of diapers. The rain was pelting down in a blinding storm, but I didn't have a choice. I had to leave you alone. I was only gone for thirty minutes, but when I returned you had fallen down in your own feces. I could barely get you back into bed. I had to bathe you, change the sheets, your diaper, and clean the carpet. It was 2:00 AM when I collapsed on my mattress. I could not sleep. You were thrashing around and moaning continuously. Your swollen stomach hurt and your body ached with every labored breath. I went into the other room to close my eyes for a few hours. But, I could not stay there either because I wouldn't have heard you calling me. I lay back down next to you at 4:00AM. My earplugs could not silence your cries. I desperately needed help with your care, but I didn't know where to turn or who to ask.

Monday, July 4th. I tried making you something to eat, but you refused. You sipped a little water or juice, but when you thought about food, you gagged and threw up. You sleep with a rubber liner under the sheets. I bought plastic runners and placed them over the carpet alongside the bed. You have to be turned every two hours in order to prevent bedsores and you must be bathed constantly. You are hooked up to an oxygen tank to assist your breathing and take several medications to control your vomiting, nausea, and pain.

Tuesday, July 5th. You asked your doctor to come to the house. When he arrived, you said, "I'm ready to die. I've had enough and want to be at home. I don't want anything else done to me." Our doctor said, "Jeff, I respect your decision and understand why. You have another option. Have you heard about Hospice? I think you and Susan are ready to have them assist you. If you are going to stay at home, they can help." We both broke down in front of him. Then he began to cry. We knew once we made the commitment for Hospice, there wouldn't be any turning back. You would not be resuscitated and we could not call 911. But on July 5th, you made the ultimate decision. Whatever time you had left, you would be in charge of your life again. Our doctor said he would make the referral tomorrow. After he left, you fell asleep. For two hours, I stood watching you as the doctor's words played over and over again in my head.

Our insurance company said they would pay for your Hospice care. There is great irony to all of this now. Though I am physically, mentally, and emotionally exhausted, I am calmer and feel stronger than I have in two years. Why should I feel this way? Is it because Hospice will help us and I am no longer alone? Is it because I trust them with your life? And why, as horrible as this time is, does a part of me want it to last? Is it because as long as you are in my life, I have a life? At 2:30 PM on Wednesday, July 6th, the Hospice social worker came to our home. She asked you how you felt and what you wanted now. Then she said to me, "Susan, can you handle this here? It will be very difficult." I said, "Yes. My husband wants it this way. I need someone two hours during the day and someone to stay with us at night." She completed her assessment and said everything would be taken care of. Home care would send someone every afternoon. The aide would bathe you and assist me. At 11:00 PM another aide would come and stay until 7:00 AM. Hospice would provide your diapers, supplies, pain medications, and order anything we needed in the future. A nurse would come in every other day and take your vital signs and assess our needs. You were treated with the respect you deserved and we had our privacy back. You were not dying in our home. You were living in it with dignity, and pride, surrounded by love.

July 20th. The pharmacy took away the walker and wheelchair. I have placed your medications and the daily supplies in a large plastic blanket box. The room is lit by candlelight and Bette Midler is singing just for you. I've rearranged the bedroom with all your favorite things. Our room smells clean and feels warm again. Though this time is chaotic, there is a sense of order and simplicity back again. I am able to schedule everyone around our Hospice help and your own needs. You only mentioned to me that you wanted to be cremated and I must use the two hours in the afternoon to make the funeral arrangements. I do not know where to begin. How do I plan a funeral for a man who's still alive? How do I bury my past when I still have a present?

July 27th. I watch you weaken daily. Your features are grotesquely deformed. You are a stranger in our bed. Your picture on the night table helps me to remember the handsome man I have loved and will soon lose. You take a few sips of water and fall back to sleep. You are comfortable and not in any pain. You are taking little medication and require oxygen occasionally. You are aware of people but barely speak. No one knows how much longer this will go on.

August 2nd. I had to write your obituary and order death certificates. It's horrible. You are still alive, but on paper you are dead. Several times today I thought you had taken your last breath. During the day, I am strong. But at night, I am afraid. Your body is stiffening, and your fingers are curled and knotted in a fist. Your skin is clammy and feels like rubber. Your ankles and feet are swollen and your eyes are dry and caked from staying open. You are gasping for air and pulling at the sheets and your clothes. Your behind is raw from the constant diaper changes. Our massage therapist comes over three times a week. He picks you up in his arms and places you in a warm bath with healing crystals. He lights candles and his soothing voice gives you pleasure.

August 8th. You continue to weaken but you are holding on. I've made the arrangements for the service, your cremation, flowers, and reception. Your doctors have come by several times to visit. They wished they could have done more. They admired your take charge attitude and courage during the past two years. The support, love, and care around you is overwhelming. It is difficult seeing your parents. I try to remain strong for them, but I want to collapse. Every night, I sit next to you for a few hours before the night aide comes. This is our precious time together. We hold hands and stare into each other's eyes. We don't need words between us. Your gestures, nods, and winks are enough. I tell you I am proud of you for doing your life your way. I thank llowing me to share it with you. You call me ╴odsend. My love, we were Godsends for each other.

August 11th. I started my journals for therapy, but now they bring me closure. I'm living through my writing. I propped you up on two pillows and wrapped your robe around you. I had never seen you looking so comfortable and relaxed. You were at peace with yourself. For the first time I said to you, "Let go, my love, let go. You proved you could do this. You took charge of your life. Let go, my love, let go."

Monday August 15th. I slept with you in my arms all night. You haven't had any liquids for two days and your breathing is shallow. Sometimes you take a breath and I think it is your last. The Strauss waltzes play continuously and candles are lit everywhere. We started our life off together in bed and we'll end it the same way. I put your gold necklace with the Chi charm, the Jewish symbol for life around your neck. I also put mine on. They were matching necklaces your father gave us when we married.

Tuesday August 16th. Your skin is clammy and cold. Your eyes are fixed open and you are staring straight ahead. Your breathing has changed. It's hard and labored. You are grasping out at everything and fighting for every breath. You are sucking in air, holding your breath, and exhaling deeply. The sounds are unimaginable and unforgettable. I stayed in bed with you while our aide slept in the vanity area on her cot. I tried to close my eyes and sleep, but couldn't. It was 3:00 AM, August 17th. I lit another candle and waited. It was 4:25AM. That was the last time I saw you alive. You waited until I fell asleep to take your last breath. I know you did not want me to see this happen. When I woke up at 4:50AM, you had died. You were staring at me just six inches away. I asked our aide to please call Hospice and tell them you had died. I called your parents. They came over immediately. We moved you to the left side of the bed, changed the sheets, removed your diaper, and straightened the room. We dressed you in your favorite Pelican T-shirt, orange Florida shorts, and thick wool socks. I had prepared several articles of clothing to be cremated with you. Your family arrived around 5:30 AM and stayed until the funeral director picked your body up at 7:00 AM. I kissed you good bye told you I loved you. I could not watch them take your body from our home.

Nobody ever knew you had starved yourself to death. It was our secret. No one would be forcing you to eat or inserting feeding tubes into you to keep you alive. There would not be another hospital room reeking of sickness and death. You controlled your death with dignity and courage. On January 11, 1969, I followed my heart, committed to love, and tried to make our marriage something special. You were my husband for twenty-five years and my one true love. On August 17, 1994, I said good-bye with the words on my lips but not in my heart. You were taken from our home, but never from my memories. I shall love you forever and be thankful for the days we had. You gave me the best years of my life. I hope I will continue to make you proud of me. You are my guardian angel and we'll always be together.

Your devoted wife and friend,

Susan Lee Mintz

Sometimes you will never know the value of a moment until it becomes a memory.

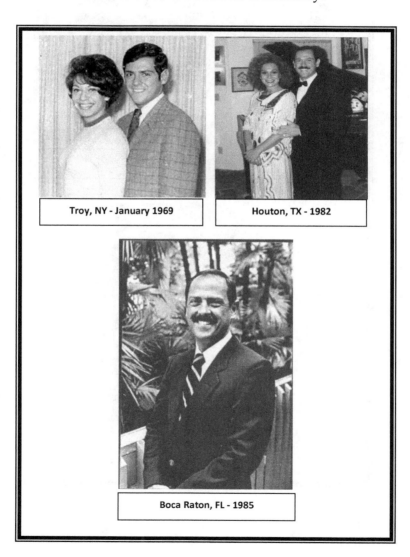

Troy, NY - January 1969

Houton, TX - 1982

Boca Raton, FL - 1985

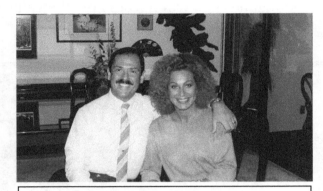

Boca Raton, FL- 1987

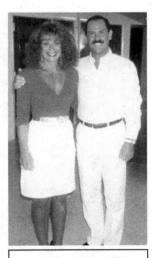

Boca Raton, FL - 1989

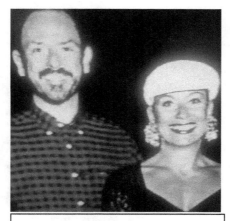

Venice, Italy - May 1994
Our last trip

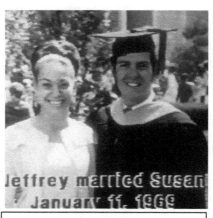

Jeffrey married Susan
January 11, 1969

Albany, NY - 1971
Master's Degree Graduation

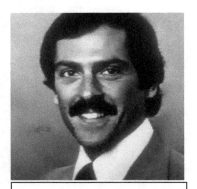

Houston, TX - 1975

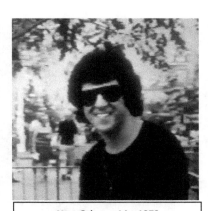

New Orleans, LA - 1973

About the Author

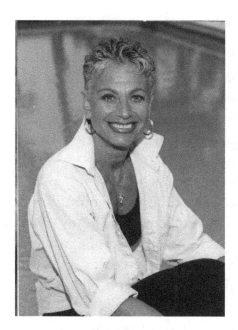

Susan Lee Mintz

About the Author

Susan Lee Mintz is a baby-boomer, motivational author, lecturer and fitness guru from Troy, New York. She currently resides in Boca Raton, Florida.

Susan is an HIV/AIDS facilitator for support groups within her area including at her church Jesus People Proclaim International Church in Deerfield Beach, Florida and at Century Village Retirement Community in Boca Raton. She serves as the Executive Director of the "I Love My Life Ministry" and the wellness center at Jesus People Proclaim. Susan has served over the years in multiple capacities and with multiple agencies to include Hospice by the Sea in Boca Raton and for 6 years was an 11th hour volunteer both at their care center and for people in their homes. Susan was a volunteer with Disaster Services of The American Red Cross, The American Association for Suicide Prevention and the Boca Raton Chamber of Commerce to name a few. Her advocacy and support of HIV/AIDS patients and families has been instrumental in helping many hurting people get through their personal stories of love and loss.

Susan's legacy includes having written several weekly motivational columns for the Boca Raton Newspaper and had been a guest speaker at the 2008 National Black HIV/AIDS Awareness Dinner (NBHAAD) held in West Palm Beach. Susan's abstinence only program was presented before the Women of Tomorrow Organization at Booker T. Washington Senior High School in Miami and throughout Florida. Susan was a volunteer with the Comprehensive AIDS Program of Palm Beach County, Real AIDS Prevention Program (RAPP), Area 9 Minority AIDS Network, and the Palm Beach County Substance Abuse Coalition (PBCSAC). Susan's lecture series entitled "YOU DON'T GET AIDS FROM LOVING SOMEBODY" has been presented throughout South Florida as she speaks openly about abstinence and testing in order to stop the spread of this deadly disease. Susan gives her testimony before youth and single ministries, in high schools, churches, synagogues, organizations, and other venues in regard to HIV/AIDS testing, education, and awareness. Susan is still an HIV/AIDS advocate for testing and believes that mandatory legislation for testing of all STD's should be put in place.

Susan is available for on/off air interviews, speaking engagements and personal appearances.

Features/ Appearances

Susan has appeared on the 700 Club with Pat
Robertson in a segment entitled "Till Death Do Us
Part" and she has also been featured on TBN's Praise
The Lord program. Susan was a contributing writer
for Prophetess Cynthia Thompson's Women You Will
Magazine which is geared to empowering, motivating,
and educating women about issues important to
women about women. Susan wrote a monthly
cooking column entitled "Cooking With Yeshua" for
the JPPIMC newsletter.

Susan legacy includes having written a weekly
motivational column for the Boca Raton Newspaper
and been a guest speaker at the 2008 National Black
HIV/AIDS Awareness Dinner (NBHAAD) held in
West Palm Beach. Susan's abstinence only program
was presented before the Women of Tomorrow
Organization at Booker T. Washington Senior High
School in Miami and Florida. Susan was a volunteer
with the Comprehensive AIDS Program of Palm
Beach County, Real AIDS Prevention Program
(RAPP), Urban 9 Minority AIDS Network, Palm
Beach County Substance Abuse Coalition (PBCSAC),
The American Foundation For Suicide Prevention,
The American Red Cross and Hospice By The Sea in

Boca Raton. Susan's lecture series entitled **"YOU DON'T GET AIDS FROM LOVING SOMEBODY"** has been presented throughout South Florida as she speaks openly about abstinence and testing in order to stop the spread of this deadly disease. Susan gives her testimony before youth and single ministries, in high schools, churches, synagogues, organizations, and other venues in regard to HIV/AIDS testing, education, and awareness. Susan is still an HIV/AIDS advocate for testing and believes that mandatory legislation for testing of all STD's should be put in place.

Susan's television appearances include: WPBF Channel 25-West Palm Beach, "Dealing With Menopause Through Weight Training"; WPTV Channel 5 -West Palm Beach-noon news live with Kelly Dunn, "Muscles, Menopause, and The Fabulous Fifties"; WRGB Channel 6 – Albany, New York, Noon News with Sue Nigra-"Bodybuilding For Baby Boomers"; WTEN Channel 10 – Albany, New York, Noon News with Tracy Egan – "Menopause and Muscles"; WNYT Channel 13 in Albany, New York in a segment on "Menopause and Bodybuilding for Baby Boomers"; Channel 23- Adelphia Cable for Lynn University in Boca Raton, Florida in the "Around Our Town" show hosted By Sid Snyder; WSVN Channel 7 in Miami, Florida for the show "Deco Drive;" "The Today Show" in Sydney, Australia; WXEL Public Television in West Palm Beach, Florida on the South Florida Today Show "Recovery After a Loved One's Loss" and "Healthy Cooking"; WPBT Public Television in Miami, Florida for Bill Moyer's Special – "On Our Own Terms" and "How Volunteering For Hospice Helped During The Recovery Process"; WPLG Channel 10 in Miami/Fort Lauderdale, Florida on "New Years Resolutions" – Sticking To An Exercise Program and "The Benefits of Weight Training During Menopause."

Her radio interviews and guest appearances include: WRMB – Moody Bible Radio–Boynton Beach, Florida- talk show host Dana Shelton; The True Christian Club of Boynton Beach Community High School; Jesus People Proclaim International Ministries Church, Boca Raton, Florida-youth ministry and congregation; WFTL-1400 Talk Radio; "The Sunday Morning Magazine Show" with Peg Browning on The Gator Radio Network, and The Coast Radio Morning Show with Terri Griffin. These interviews included questions concerning her marriage and AIDS. Daily newspapers and monthly magazines have printed articles about Susan including those appearing in: *The Jewish Star Times, Natural Awakenings, The Boca Raton*

News, The South Florida Sun-Sentinel, The Happy Times Newspaper, and Vital Signs Magazine (South Florida's #1 Resource Guide to Nurses and Health Care Professionals) in a question and answer column titled "The Benefits of Bodybuilding During Menopause." She also wrote a column in the*Boca Raton News* titled "With a Hospice Heart," and serves as a contributing writer and columnist for *Natural MuscleMagazine, Michael Body Scenes Magazine,* and*The Boca Del Mar Newsletter.*

Susan has spoken at the following Bookstores in South Florida about her lecture series entitled "You Don't Get AIDS From Loving Somebody." Borders Books and Music, Barnes and Noble Bookstores, and Liberties Books in Mizner Park and Ft. Lauderdale . Her speaking engagements for non-profit organizations in South Florida include: Hadassah, ORT, City of Hope , Women's Clubs, Condominium Associations, Civic Groups, BocaCares, Professional Women's Organizations, Hospice By The Sea, The Comprehensive AIDS Program of Palm Beach County and the Adolph & Rose Levis Jewish Community Center (JCC).

Susan was featured as a guest lecturer and keynote speaker at the following events: North Broward

Regional Medical Center-Health Fair, Expos, and Seminars; Women Health Fairs and Seminars at the Boca Raton Community Hospital, West Boca Community Hospital, CAP, and the JCC. The Comprehensive AIDS Program has featured Susan as a keynote speaker for its annual Walk For Life in West Palm Beach, Florida and at numerous fundraisers where she signs her cookbook, "Safe Sex Never Tasted So Good." Hospice by the Sea in Boca Raton has her on its Speakers' Bureau. Susan represents Hospice at health fairs, educational seminars, local hospitals, and at events like the Boca Expo, The Delray Affair, workshops, and vending booths at local malls.

PERSONAL BACKGROUND

Once a professional dental hygienist, Susan married her elementary-school sweetheart, **Jeffrey**, at the age of 22. Their marriage was passionate and full of ups and downs with the surprising revelation that Jeffrey was bi-sexual. Her enduring love and unconditional acceptance for Jeffrey during this difficult period never wavered. For 25 years, Susan kept her commitment to their marriage. In June 1992, Jeffrey was diagnosed with AIDS. She rallied with him in the fight for his life. On August 17, 1994 , Jeffrey passed away in the privacy of their home with the help of hospice. Jeffrey's death left Susan searching for comfort and support which she later found through writing, exercise, cooking, and her faith.

Susan's proclivity towards nutrition developed into a penchant for cooking. She began cooking up a storm relying upon her humor and motivational attitude while pleasing palates everywhere. Her recipes were healthy, creative, easy-to-prepare and flavorful with off-color and shockingly unique names. She penned these and other recipes into a renowned cookbook titled "Safe Sex Never Tasted So Good" with partial proceeds benefiting non-profit organizations. Cooking enabled Susan to make a positive and immediate impact in the lives of others through nutrition.

Susan pursued her cooking with passion and was forced to further challenge her culinary skills when she began weight training. Her discipline motivated many people who she influenced and taught through personal training in the South Florida area. When Susan isn't writing, cooking, or working out, she contributed her time and efforts through her volunteer work and community involvement. At Hospice by the Sea, she served as an 11th hour volunteer–one who is called when a patient's death is imminent-and educates others about AIDS through the Comprehensive AIDS Program (CAP) of Palm Beach County, Florida.

Other Books & Contact Info

Contact Susan

www.SusanMintz.com

Email: smintz7179@aol.com **Phone:** 561-271-1879

Facebook: Susan Mintz

Committed to Love

A Woman's Journey through Love and Loss

Book Ordering Information:

$26.95 Hardback

$22.95 Paperback // $12ea for Bulk orders of 25+

$9.95 eBook

And I Held their Hands with a Hospice Heart

- Stories of Hope, Faith, Love and Loss

Book Ordering Information:

$22.95 Paperback // $12ea for Bulk orders of 25+

$9.95 eBook

Order at **www.PurposePublishing.com**

Leave comments at Susan **www.SusanMintz.com**

Coming Soon

Cooking with Yeshua

CPSIA information can be obtained
at www.ICGtesting.com
Printed in the USA
BVHW042219210319
543422BV00015BA/168/P